DRCOG: PRACTICE MCQs AND OSCEs:
HOW TO PASS FIRST TIME

I dedicate this book to my husband, William,
and to my three daughters, Olivia, Emily and Henrietta

DRCOG: PRACTICE MCQs AND OSCEs: HOW TO PASS FIRST TIME
THREE COMPLETE MCQ PRACTICE EXAMS (180 MCQs)
THREE COMPLETE OSCE PRACTICE PAPERS (60 QUESTIONS)
DETAILED ANSWERS AND TIPS

By

Una F. Coales
BA MD FRCS (ED) FRCS (OTO) DRCOG
Senior House Officer
Department of Obstetrics and Gynaecology
King's College Hospital
Denmark Hill
London, UK

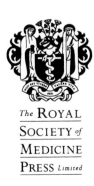

The ROYAL
SOCIETY of
MEDICINE
PRESS Limited

British Library Cataloguing in Publication Data
A catalogue record for this book is available from the British Library

ISBN: 1–85315–506–3

Typeset by Phoenix Photosetting, Chatham, Kent

Printed in Great Britain by Bell and Bain Ltd, Glasgow

Contents

Preface

The Diploma of the Royal College of Obstetricians and Gynaecologists (DRCOG) examination consists of 60 multiple choice questions (MCQs) and 22 six-minute objective structured clinical examination stations (OSCEs), of which two are rest stations. The one-day examination is designed for general practice trainees, ideally with 6 months experience in obstetrics and gynaecology at the senior house officer grade.

This book presents three complete DRCOG MCQ and OSCE circuits and encompasses all the possible MCQ and OSCE topics that can and have been asked in the DRCOG examination. Take my advice. Read, understand and digest this book thoroughly, and you will pass the DRCOG examination first time, as I did.

Una F. Coales
September 2001

Acknowledgements

I thank the Department of Obstetrics and Gynaecology, King's College Hospital, London, and, in particular, the following individuals for their invaluable support and contribution to the content of this book:

Mr Davor Jurkovic MD, MRCOG (Consultant in Obstetrics and Gynaecology).

Mr Anthony Davies MRCOG (Consultant in Obstetrics and Gynaecology).

Dr Janine Elson DFFP, MRCOG (Specialist Registrar in Obstetrics and Gynaecology).

Dr Usha Kumar MRCOG (Specialist Registrar in Obstetrics and Gynaecology).

Dr Rehan Salim MBBS (Research Fellow in Obstetrics and Gynaecology).

Recommended texts and references

Chamberlain G. & Hamilton-Fairly D. (1999) *Lecture Notes on Obstetrics and Gynaecology*. Blackwell, Oxford.

Collier J.A.B. *et al.* (1994) *Oxford Handbook of Clinical Specialties*, 3rd edn. Oxford University Press, Oxford.

Fauci A. *et al.* (1997) *Harrison's Principles of Internal Medicine*, 14th edn. McGraw-Hill, New York.

Glasier A. *et al.* (2000) *Handbook of Family Planning and Reproductive Healthcare*, 4th edn. Churchill Livingstone, London.

Hacker N.F. *et al.* (1998) *Essentials of Obstetrics and Gynaecology*, 3rd edn. W.B. Saunders, Philadelphia.

Jawetz E. *et al.* (1987) *Review of Medical Microbiology*, 17th edn. Appleton & Lange, Connecticut.

Royal Pharmaceutical Society of Great Britain (2001) *British National Formulary*. British Medical Association, London.

Rymer J. *et al.* (1998) *Preparation and Revision for the DRCOG*, 2nd edn. Churchill Livingstone, London.

Department of Health (1998) *Why Mothers Die – Report on Confidential Enquiries into Maternal Deaths in the United Kingdom 1994–1996*. Department of Health, London.

DRCOG MCQs for Circuit A
Questions

1. **In which circumstances is rhesus immunization required in a rhesus-negative mother?**
   A. Following amniocentesis.
   B. After delivery of a rhesus-negative baby.
   C. After a threatened miscarriage at 10 weeks' gestation.
   D. After termination of pregnancy at 8 weeks' gestation.
   E. After a spontaneous miscarriage at 8 weeks' gestation.

2. **Endometrial cancer is associated with:**
   A. Combined oral contraceptive pills.
   B. Premarin use in the postmenopausal woman with a uterus.
   C. Early menopause.
   D. Obesity.
   E. Multiple pregnancy.

3. **Turner's syndrome is associated with:**
   A. Oestrogen sensitivity.
   B. Co-arctation of the aorta.
   C. Webbed neck.
   D. Short stature.
   E. Increase in follicle-stimulating hormone.

4. **Routine blood tests taken in the Antenatal Clinic include:**
   A. Human immunodeficiency virus (HIV).
   B. Hepatitis A.
   C. Haemoglobin electrophoresis in pregnant women from India.
   D. Full blood count.
   E. Clotting studies.

5. **Laparoscopic sterilization:**
   A. Reversible in 70% of cases with the use of a microscope.
   B. Lower failure rate if performed at the time of Caesarean section.
   C. 20% risk of postoperative ectopic pregnancy.
   D. Fewer complications than a vasectomy.
   E. Failure rate of 1 in 100.

6. **Increased serum human chorionic gonadotrophin (hCG) is associated with:**
   A. Choriocarcinoma.
   B. Hyperemesis gravidarum.
   C. Hepatoma.
   D. Ovarian carcinoma.
   E. Hydatidiform mole.

7. Oligohydramnios is associated with:
   A. Pulmonary hypoplasia.
   B. Oesophageal atresia.
   C. Spina bifida.
   D. Renal agenesis.
   E. Anencephaly.

8. Cervical smear may suggest the diagnosis of:
   A. Adenomyosis.
   B. Bacterial vaginosis.
   C. *Trichomonas vaginalis*.
   D. Cervical intraepithelial neoplasia (CIN).
   E. Invasive carcinoma of the cervix.

9. Mirena coil:
   A. Contains levonorgestrel.
   B. Controls menorrhagia.
   C. Needs to be changed every 5 years.
   D. Safe in women with a history of pelvic inflammatory disease (PID).
   E. Increases the absolute risk of ectopic pregnancy.

10. Puberty:
    A. Associated with anovular cycles.
    B. Onset of pubic hair occurs before breast bud development.
    C. Begins with the first menstrual cycle.
    D. May be associated with cervical ectropion.
    E. May be associated with dysfunctional uterine bleeding.

11. Post-coital bleeding can occur with:
    A. Cervical polyp.
    B. Cervical intraepithelial neoplasia (CIN).
    C. *Trichomonas vaginalis* infection.
    D. Cervical ectropion.
    E. Endometrial carcinoma.

12. Deep dyspareunia can occur with:
    A. Pelvic inflammatory disease (PID).
    B. Vaginismus.
    C. Bartholin's cyst.
    D. *Herpes genitalis* infection.
    E. Endometriosis.

13. **Intermenstrual bleeding may be associated with:**
    A. Fibroids.
    B. Polycystic ovarian syndrome.
    C. Carcinoma of the cervix.
    D. Combined oral contraceptives.
    E. Intrauterine copper device.

14. **Pearl Index:**
    A. Defined as the failure rate per 100 woman-years.
    B. 0.5% for use of the combined oral contraceptive (coc) pill.
    C. 2% for the use of a condom with a spermicide.
    D. 1% for the progesterone-only pill.
    E. 1% for the intrauterine system (IUS).

15. **Syntometrine:**
    A. Composed of 5 units oxytocin and 500 mcg ergonometrine maleate.
    B. Contraindicated in the second stage of labour.
    C. Given intramuscularly before surgical evacuation of the uterus in an incomplete abortion.
    D. Known side-effects of nausea and dizziness.
    E. Given with or after delivery of the shoulders in the third stage of labour.

16. **Apgar score:**
    A. Taken at 1 and 5 minutes after birth.
    B. Assesses heart rate, respiratory rate, colour, muscle tone and reflex/irritability.
    C. Named after Dr Virginia Apgar.
    D. Neonate assessed at 1 minute with a heart rate of 90 bpm, a respiratory rate of 20 breaths per minute, that grimaces and moves all limbs freely with blue extremities has an Apgar score = 6.
    E. Neonate with a heart rate of 90 bpm and no respirations should have face mask resuscitation.

17. **Appropriate investigations for a 32-year-old woman 5 days post-emergency Caesarean section who now presents with per vagina bleeding and passage of blood clots include:**
    A. Transvaginal ultrasound scan.
    B. Full blood count.
    C. Vaginal swab for microscopy and culture.
    D. Blood for group and save.
    E. Clotting studies.

18. Causes of preterm labour include:
    A. Chorio-amnionitis.
    B. Polyhydramnios.
    C. Cervical incompetence.
    D. Peritonitis.
    E. Pyelonephritis.

19. Causes of pruritus vulvae include:
    A. Genital prolapse.
    B. Hyperthyroidism.
    C. Diabetes mellitus.
    D. *Herpes genitalis*.
    E. Leukoplakia.

20. Complications of pre-eclampsia include:
    A. Intrauterine growth retardation (IUGR).
    B. Renal failure.
    C. Thrombocytopaenia.
    D. Cerebrovascular accident.
    E. Fetal death.

21. The following are neonatal risks in a mother with IDDM:
    A. Hyaline membrane disease.
    B. Congenital heart disease.
    C. Hypermagnesaemia.
    D. Shoulder dystocia.
    E. Sacral agenesis.

22. The following are obstetric risks to a pregnant mother with IDDM:
    A. Pre-eclampsia.
    B. Preterm labour.
    C. Oligohydramnios.
    D. Recurrent miscarriage.
    E. Postpartum haemorrhage.

23. Maternal causes of intrauterine growth retardation (IUGR) include:
    A. Alcohol intake.
    B. Diabetes mellitus.
    C. Placenta abruptio.
    D. Hypertension.
    E. Renal impairment.

24. **Causes of symmetric intrauterine growth retardation (IUGR) include:**
    A. Toxoplasmosis.
    B. Down's syndrome.
    C. Twins.
    D. Rubella.
    E. Cytomegalovirus infection.

25. **Signs and symptoms of polycystic ovarian syndrome include:**
    A. Bulimia.
    B. Acne.
    C. Oligomenorrhoea.
    D. Infertility.
    E. Amenorrhoea.

26. **Side-effects of clomiphene citrate include:**
    A. Visual disturbances.
    B. Hot flushes.
    C. Intermenstrual spotting.
    D. Weight gain.
    E. Hair loss.

27. **Causes of neonatal jaundice within the first 24 hours of life include:**
    A. ABO incompatibility.
    B. Hypothyroidism.
    C. Physiological.
    D. Polycythaemia.
    E. Rhesus incompatibility.

28. **Causes of prolonged neonatal jaundice over 2 weeks include:**
    A. Hypopituitarism.
    B. Galactosaemia.
    C. Breast-feeding.
    D. Cystic fibrosis.
    E. Neonatal hepatitis.

29. **Contraindications to oestrogen replacement therapy include:**
    A. Undiagnosed vaginal bleeding.
    B. Chronic impaired liver function.
    C. Migrainous headaches.
    D. Pre-existing seizures.
    E. Endometrial cancer.

30. **Causes of dysmenorrhoea include:**
    A. Endometriosis.
    B. IUD.
    C. Pelvic inflammatory disease (PID).
    D. Fibroids.
    E. Polycystic ovarian disease.

31. **Malignant vulval carcinoma:**
    A. Mostly occurs in the 75–80-year age group.
    B. May be associated with lichen sclerosus.
    C. May be associated with human papilloma virus (HPV).
    D. Stage II is treated with radical vulvectomy and bilateral groin node dissection.
    E. Nodes that can become involved include external iliac, femoral and superficial inguinal.

32. **Stage Ia cervical carcinoma:**
    A. Penetrates the basement membrane into the stroma up to 3 mm.
    B. Micro-invasive.
    C. Diagnosed by cone biopsy of the cervix.
    D. Treated by radical hysterectomy and bilateral pelvic lymphadenopathy.
    E. May be symptomless.

33. **Meconium staining of the amniotic fluid may be associated with:**
    A. Umbilical cord compression.
    B. Intrauterine growth retardation (IUGR).
    C. Uterine hypertonicity.
    D. Post-term pregnancy.
    E. Polyhydramnios.

34. **Human papilloma virus (HPV):**
    A. Associated with the presence of koilocytes on a cervical smear.
    B. HPV16 and 18 are associated with cervical neoplasia.
    C. May appear as exophytic warts or flat condylomata on the cervix.
    D. Associated with genital warts.
    E. Systemic absorption of podophyllin used may cause peripheral neuropathy.

35. **Intrauterine contraceptive device:**
    A. Increases the relative risk of ectopic pregnancy.
    B. Contraindicated in Wilson's disease.
    C. Contraindicated in congenital or rheumatic heart disease.
    D. Replaced every 5 years.
    E. Controls menorrhagia.

36. **Bartholin's glands:**
    A. Bartholin's abscess may be due to *Gonococcus* infection.
    B. Bartholin's abscess is treated adequately by marsupialization.
    C. Also called the minor vestibular glands.
    D. Duct opens into the vestibule at the junction of the labium minora and the hymen between the anterior two-thirds and the posterior one-third.
    E. Bartholin's abscess may be due to *Escherichia coli* infection.

37. **Vulval ulcers may be due to:**
    A. Lymphogranuloma inguinale.
    B. *Herpes simplex*.
    C. Tuberculosis.
    D. Behçet's disease.
    E. Chancroid.

38. **Ectopic pregnancy:**
    A. Risk factor includes the intrauterine device (IUD).
    B. Occurs in 1 in 200 pregnancies.
    C. Classically presents with shoulder tip pain.
    D. Never presents with bilateral lower abdominal pain.
    E. May be treated with injection of methotrexate into the unruptured ectopic.

39. **Malignant ovarian tumours include:**
    A. Clear cell tumour.
    B. Brenner tumour.
    C. Granulosa cell tumour.
    D. Dysgerminoma.
    E. Krukenberg.

40. **Causes of vaginal discharge in pregnancy include:**
    A. *Trichomonas vaginalis*.
    B. Bacterial vaginosis.
    C. *Herpes genitalis*.
    D. *Chlamydia*.
    E. Toxoplasmosis.

41. **Appropriate forms of contraception after delivery for a mother who plans to breast-feed include:**
    A. Implanon.
    B. Progestogen-only pill.
    C. Depo-Provera.
    D. Intrauterine contraceptive device (IUCD).
    E. Combined oral contraceptive pill.

42. **According to the Report on Confidential Enquiries into Maternal Deaths in the UK, 1994–1996:**
    A. 11.5 ectopic pregnancies per 1000 pregnancies.
    B. Maternal death rate per 1000 ectopic pregnancies was 1.4.
    C. Direct abortion death rate per 1 million estimated pregnancies was 1.0.
    D. Reported maternal death rate per 100 000 maternities was 12.2.
    E. Leading cause of direct maternal death was due to thrombosis and thromboembolism.

43. **Tuberculosis of the genital tract:**
    A. Tuberculous salpingitis often results in female sterility.
    B. May be diagnosed by endometrial biopsy.
    C. Genital tuberculosis often occurs in older women with half being postmenopausal.
    D. Can result in congenital tuberculosis if untreated during pregnancy.
    E. Diagnosis is made by culture of acid-fast bacilli.

44. **An estimated fundal height that is large for dates based on LMP may be associated with:**
    A. Twin pregnancy.
    B. Gestational diabetes mellitus.
    C. Molar pregnancy.
    D. 35-day menstrual cycle.
    E. Multiparity.

45. **Uterine retroversion:**
    A. Found in 20% of women.
    B. Fixed retroversion may result in dystocia in labour.
    C. Fixed retroversion may result in urinary retention in pregnancy.
    D. In pregnancy, the retroverted uterus grows out of the bony pelvis by 14 weeks.
    E. In pregnancy, the retroverted uterus may result in upward displacement of the bladder into the abdomen.

46. **Human immunodeficiency virus (HIV) is transmitted through:**
    A. Urine.
    B. Blood.
    C. Semen.
    D. Breast milk.
    E. Saliva.

47. **Congenital hip dislocation:**
    A. More common in females than in males.
    B. Can be detected at birth.
    C. Often painful.
    D. Will result in a palpable 'clunk' (Ortolani's sign) when the hips are slowly abducted from a 90° flexed position.
    E. May be associated with breech presentation.

48. **Moniliasis is a complication of:**
    A. Diabetes mellitus.
    B. Pregnancy.
    C. Immunosuppressive therapy.
    D. Prolonged antibiotic use.
    E. Steroid therapy.

49. **Salpingitis is associated with:**
    A. Sterility.
    B. Ectopic pregnancy.
    C. Tuberculosis.
    D. Gonococcal infection.
    E. Retrograde infection.

50. **Vomiting in late pregnancy may be associated with:**
    A. Hydatidiform mole.
    B. Hiatal hernia.
    C. Pre-eclampsia.
    D. Appendicitis.
    E. Pyelonephritis.

51. **Differential diagnosis for postmenopausal bleeding includes:**
    A. Carcinoma of the cervix.
    B. Adenomyosis.
    C. Endometrial polyp.
    D. Atrophic vaginitis.
    E. Endometrial carcinoma.

52. **Causes of proteinuria in pregnancy include:**
    A. Acute pyelonephritis.
    B. Abruptio placenta without pre-eclampsia.
    C. Chronic glomerulonephritis.
    D. Diabetic nephropathy.
    E. Uncomplicated essential hypertension.

53. **Endometrial hyperplasia is characteristically associated with:**
    A. Essential hypertension.
    B. Polycystic ovarian disease.
    C. Premature menopause.
    D. Hypothyroidism.
    E. Unopposed oestrogen therapy.

54. **Diabetes mellitus in pregnancy is associated with:**
    A. Recurrent urinary tract infections.
    B. Pre-eclampsia.
    C. Sacral agenesis.
    D. Increase in insulin requirement during pregnancy.
    E. Prematurity.

55. **External cephalic version:**
    A. Used to convert a breech presentation to cephalic presentation.
    B. Not contraindicated if there is a prior Caesarean section scar.
    C. Can cause premature labour.
    D. Contraindicated in hypertension.
    E. Can be performed after 33 weeks' gestation in a rhesus-negative mother.

56. **Breech presentation:**
    A. Flexed breech is more common in multipara.
    B. Associated with an anthropoid pelvis.
    C. Kielland forceps are used after coning of the head.
    D. Associated with a bitrochanteric diameter of 10 cm.
    E. More common in prematurity.

57. **Drugs that may be used in pregnancy include:**
    A. Erythromycin.
    B. Streptomycin.
    C. Metronidazole.
    D. Trimethoprim.
    E. Tetracycline.

58. **Endometrial carcinoma is associated with:**
    A. Endometriosis.
    B. Polycystic ovarian disease.
    C. Previous anovulatory cycles.
    D. Human papilloma virus (HPV) 16 and 18.
    E. Dysfunctional uterine bleeding.

59. **Causes of menorrhagia include:**
    A. Pelvic inflammatory disease.
    B. Endometriosis.
    C. Hyperprolactinaemia.
    D. Idiopathic thrombocytopaenic purpura.
    E. Hyperthyroidism.

60. **Causes of primary postpartum haemorrhage include:**
    A. Hydramnios.
    B. Syntocinon drip in the first stage of labour.
    C. Prolonged labour.
    D. Abruptio placenta.
    E. Pre-eclampsia.

DRCOG MCQs for Circuit B
Questions

1. *Chlamydia trachomatis*:
   A. Gram-positive intracellular bacterium.
   B. Can cause blindness.
   C. Treated with doxycycline.
   D. Cause of salpingitis.
   E. Can cause perihepatitis.

2. *Neisseria gonorrhoea*:
   A. Gram-negative diplococcus bacterium.
   B. Infects the baby during childbirth.
   C. Causes ophthalmia neonatorum.
   D. Causes urethritis.
   E. Can cause perihepatitis.

3. **Causes of transverse lie include:**
   A. Arcuate uterus.
   B. Polyhydramnios.
   C. Fibroids.
   D. Placenta praevia.
   E. Twins.

4. **Causes of prolonged labour include:**
   A. Cephalopelvic disproportion.
   B. Android pelvis.
   C. Brow presentation.
   D. Persistent occipitoposterior position.
   E. Uterine inertia.

5. **Secondary dysmenorrhoea:**
   A. May precede menstruation.
   B. Usually associated with organic disease.
   C. Occurs shortly after menarche.
   D. Means painful menstruation.
   E. May be psychosexual in aetiology.

6. **An infant with jaundice 6 hours after delivery may have:**
   A. Physiological jaundice.
   B. Rhesus incompatibility.
   C. Atresia of the bile ducts.
   D. Meconium ileus.
   E. ABO incompatibility.

7. **Anovulatory cycles are associated with:**
   A. Infertility.
   B. Dysfunctional uterine bleeding.
   C. Irregular duration.
   D. Climacteric.
   E. Increased risk of endometrial carcinoma.

8. **Endometriosis characteristically causes:**
   A. Intestinal stricture.
   B. Painful laparotomy scar.
   C. Secondary dysmenorrhoea.
   D. Deep dyspareunia.
   E. Mittelschmerz.

9. **Vesicovaginal fistula may be associated with:**
   A. Increased incidence of urinary tract infections.
   B. Continuous wetting.
   C. Bladder distension.
   D. Carcinoma of the cervix.
   E. Faecal incontinence.

10. **Secondary amenorrhoea is associated with:**
   A. Anorexia nervosa.
   B. Leiomyoma.
   C. Thyrotoxicosis.
   D. Endometriosis.
   E. Menopause.

11. **Cryptomenorrhoea in a 15-year-old girl is associated with:**
   A. Short stature.
   B. Absence of secondary sexual characteristics.
   C. Chromosomal abnormality.
   D. Atresia of the Müllerian ducts.
   E. Imperforate hymen.

12. **Per vagina (PV) bleed in an 8-year-old girl may be associated with:**
   A. Sarcoma botyroides.
   B. Urethral prolapse.
   C. Granulosa theca cell tumour.
   D. Dysgerminoma.
   E. Adrenal tumour.

13. **Laparoscopic sterilization:**
   A. Reversible in 70% of cases if performed microscopically.
   B. Higher failure rate if performed at the time of Caesarean section.
   C. Associated with ectopic pregnancy as a late complication.
   D. Mortality rate of 1 in 10 000.
   E. Failure rate of < 0.5% in the first year.

14. **Adenomyosis.**
    A. Means endometriosis within the myometrium.
    B. Presents with secondary dysmenorrhoea.
    C. Often associated with amenorrhoea.
    D. May occur within a uterine fibroid.
    E. Predisposes to myometrial leiomyosarcoma.

15. **The following factors increase the success of trial of scar:**
    A. One normal vaginal delivery after the first Caesarean section.
    B. Elective Caesarean section at the previous pregnancy.
    C. Emergency Caesarean section at the previous pregnancy.
    D. Non-recurrent indication (i.e. fetal distress) for the previous Caesarean section.
    E. Recurrent indication for the previous Caesarean section.

16. **Postpartum deep venous thromboembolism is associated with:**
    A. Low-grade pyrexia.
    B. Unilateral lower leg oedema.
    C. Blood group O.
    D. Multiparity.
    E. Increased maternal age (> 40 years).

17. **Drugs that can be safely administered during pregnancy include:**
    A. Sodium valproate.
    B. Propranolol.
    C. ACE inhibitors.
    D. Carbamazepine.
    E. NSAIDs.

18. **A pregnancy associated with an anencephalic fetus is associated with:**
    A. Polyhydramnios.
    B. Prolonged gestation.
    C. Fetal adrenal hypoplasia.
    D. Fetus is commonly female.
    E. Dystocia.

19. **Recognized sequelae of salpingitis include:**
    A. Ectopic pregnancy.
    B. Infertility.
    C. Tubo-ovarian abscess.
    D. Endometriosis.
    E. Superficial thrombophlebitis.

20. **Post-coital bleeding may be caused by:**
    A.   Adenomyosis.
    B.   Atrophic vaginitis.
    C.   Cervical ectropion.
    D.   Cervical polyp.
    E.   Carcinoma of the cervix.

21. **Management of an HIV-positive pregnant mother includes:**
    A.   Caesarean section delivery in all cases.
    B.   Zidovudine oral therapy to the infant for a minimum of 6 weeks.
    C.   Measurement of the CD4 count and viral load.
    D.   Avoidance of breast-feeding.
    E.   Zidovudine oral therapy to the mother from week 14 of gestation to labour and then intravenous therapy during labour and delivery.

22. **Complications of hysterectomy include:**
    A.   Injury to the ureter.
    B.   Atelectasis.
    C.   Uterovaginal fistula.
    D.   Thrombophlebitis.
    E.   Pelvic abscess.

23. **Osteoporosis:**
    A.   Oestrogen increases bone mass.
    B.   Raloxifene is licensed for the prevention and treatment of spinal osteoporosis and may reduce the risk of breast cancer.
    C.   Characterized by a decrease in the number and size of the trabeculae of cancellous bone.
    D.   One in two women over 70 years will have an osteoporotic-related fracture.
    E.   Bisphosphonates decrease the risk of vertebral fractures in the postmenopausal woman.

24. **Risk factors for osteoporosis include:**
    A.   Cigarette smoking.
    B.   Early menopause.
    C.   Family history.
    D.   Excess alcohol intake.
    E.   Lack of physical activity.

25. **Disseminated intracellular coagulopathy is associated with:**
    A. Abruptio placentae.
    B. Amniotic fluid embolism.
    C. Intrauterine fetal demise.
    D. Severe pre-eclampsia.
    E. Transfusion reaction.

26. **Hyperemesis gravidarum:**
    A. Does not recur in subsequent pregnancies.
    B. Metoclopramide may induce oculogyric crises.
    C. May be associated with multiple pregnancy.
    D. May be associated with a hydatidiform mole.
    E. May be associated with jaundice.

27. **Down's syndrome is associated with:**
    A. Duodenal atresia.
    B. Chromosomal translocation, which occurs in 20% of cases.
    C. Overall incidence of 1 in 650 live births.
    D. Approximate risk of an affected child of 1 in 365 at a maternal age of 35 years.
    E. Hypotonia.

28. **Use of the contraceptive diaphragm requires:**
    A. Refitting if the woman loses or gains 3 kg in weight.
    B. Refitting after a miscarriage.
    C. Retention for 6 hours after sexual intercourse.
    D. Addition of spermicide for increased efficacy.
    E. Removal within 30 hours of continued use.

29. **Face presentation may be associated with:**
    A. Anecephaly.
    B. Multiple pregnancy.
    C. Polyhydramnios.
    D. Maternal congenital hip dislocation.
    E. Fibroids.

30. **Fibroids may be associated with:**
    A. Intermenstrual bleeding.
    B. Infertility.
    C. Urinary retention.
    D. Dyspareunia.
    E. Anaemia.

31. **Asymptomatic bacteriuria in pregnancy may be associated with:**
    A. *Escherichia coli* infection.
    B. > 100,000 bacteria ml^{-1} urine.
    C. 30% risk of acute pyelonephritis in pregnancy.
    D. Preterm labour.
    E. *Proteus mirabilis* infection.

32. **Dyspareunia may be associated with:**
    A. Climacteric.
    B. Pelvic inflammatory disease (PID).
    C. Endometriosis.
    D. Endometrial carcinoma.
    E. Cervical intraepithelial neoplasia (CIN).

33. **Risk factors for respiratory distress syndrome (RDS) include:**
    A. Diabetic mother.
    B. Birth weight at term < 10th centile.
    C. Born before 32 weeks' gestation.
    D. Steroid administration between 28 and 32 weeks' gestation.
    E. Lecithin/sphingomyelin ratio of < 2 and no phosphatidylglycerol.

34. **In normal pregnancy:**
    A. Peripheral resistance decreases.
    B. Cervical cytology is associated with high false-positives.
    C. 100 mg elemental iron and 350 mcg (micrograms) folic acid are recommended as daily supplements.
    D. Haemoglobin may fall by 1 g dl^{-1} due to relative haemodilution.
    E. Increased resistance to insulin.

35. **In a newborn:**
    A. Bowel is sterile.
    B. Ductus arteriosus closes immediately after delivery.
    C. Physiological jaundice occurs between 6 and 8 days.
    D. Pulse rate is 90–100 bpm.
    E. 1 mg vitamin K is administered intramuscularly to prevent haemorrhagic disease of the newborn.

36. ***Trichomonas vaginalis*:**
    A. Can be diagnosed by exfoliative cytology.
    B. Responds to metronidazole.
    C. May present with strawberry patches on the cervix.
    D. Flagellated protozoon.
    E. May infect the Bartholin's glands.

37. **Cervical erosion:**
    A. Cause of intermenstrual bleeding.
    B. Covered by squamous epithelium.
    C. May be treated by cryosurgery.
    D. Commonly occurs in pregnancy.
    E. May be diagnosed by cervical cytology.

38. **Risk factors for pregnancy-induced hypertension include:**
    A. Multiple pregnancy.
    B. Multiparity.
    C. Maternal smoking in pregnancy.
    D. Hydatidiform mole.
    E. Consanguinous marriage.

39. **Forceps delivery is indicated in:**
    A. Cord prolapse with the cervix fully dilated.
    B. Failure to progress in the second stage with the head in the OP position.
    C. A mother with cardiac disease to avoid strenuous pushing.
    D. Cases of fetal hypoxia with the membranes intact.
    E. Delivery of the head in breech presentation.

40. **Endometrial carcinoma:**
    A. Occurs in an older age group than cervical carcinoma.
    B. More common than cervical carcinoma.
    C. Usually a squamous cell carcinoma.
    D. Stage Ic is characterized by carcinoma confined to the uterine body with invasion of more than half of the myometrium.
    E. Stage II is characterized by carcinoma involving the body of the uterus and the cervix.

41. **First stage of labour is shortened by:**
    A. Artificial rupture of the membranes.
    B. Forceps intervention.
    C. Caesarean section.
    D. Ergometrine intravenously.
    E. Oxytocin drip.

42. **Treatment of postpartum haemorrhage (PPH) includes:**
    A. Uterine packing.
    B. Vaginal packing.
    C. Intravenous ergotamine.
    D. Uterine exploration.
    E. Laparotomy.

43. **Ectopic pregnancy:**
    A. Most implant in the ampulla.
    B. Higher recurrence rate.
    C. Decidual endometrium is shed.
    D. May present with shoulder tip pain.
    E. Blood loss may be dark or 'prune juice' in colour.

44. **Unstable lie in late pregnancy may be associated with:**
    A. Bicornuate uterus.
    B. Uterine fibroids.
    C. Intrauterine growth retardation (IUGR).
    D. Placenta praevia.
    E. Indication for hospital admission before term.

45. **Puerperal psychosis is associated with:**
    A. 1 in 500 births.
    B. Severe depression.
    C. Suicidal tendencies.
    D. Delusions.
    E. Requires compulsory admission with the baby if possible.

46. **Haemoglobin < 10 g dl^{-1} in pregnancy:**
    A. Associated with an increased risk of urinary tract infection.
    B. Recognized side-effect of anti-epileptic drugs.
    C. Readily responds to oral iron supplements.
    D. Increases the risk of postpartum haemorrhage.
    E. Common in sickle cell trait.

47. **Recognized signs of deep venous thrombosis (DVT) include:**
    A. Low-grade pyrexia.
    B. More common in the left leg than in the right.
    C. Coexistent varicose veins.
    D. Positive Homan's sign.
    E. Local calf tenderness.

48. **Treatment of polycystic ovary syndrome includes:**
    A. Dianette.
    B. Clomiphene.
    C. Zoladex.
    D. Danazol.
    E. Tranexamic acid.

49. **Polycystic ovarian syndrome is associated with:**
    A. LH/FSH ratio > 3 during the first week of the cycle.
    B. Increased testosterone.
    C. Absent menses.
    D. Infertility.
    E. Increased risk of endometrial carcinoma.

50. **Primary postpartum haemorrhage:**
    A. Involves blood loss > 500 ml within 24 hours of delivery.
    B. Causes a greater maternal mortality rate than antepartum haemorrhage.
    C. May be associated with eclampsia.
    D. May be associated with high parity.
    E. May be associated with amniotic fluid embolus.

51. **Cytology of a cervical smear may diagnose:**
    A. Bacterial vaginosis.
    B. Endometrial carcinoma.
    C. HSV.
    D. HPV.
    E. *Chlamydia.*

52. **Contraindications for the use of the intrauterine contraceptive device (IUCD) include:**
    A. Submucous fibroids.
    B. Bicornuate uterus.
    C. Valvular heart implant.
    D. Cervical ectropion.
    E. Subserous fibroids.

53. **Differential diagnosis for a 17-year-old woman complaining of lower abdominal pain and irregular vaginal bleeding includes:**
    A. Pelvic inflammatory disease (PID).
    B. Uterine sarcoma.
    C. Ectopic pregnancy.
    D. Benign cystic teratoma.
    E. Metropathia haemorrhagica.

54. **Vulvar dystrophy:**
    A. Presents with pruritus.
    B. Can be premalignant.
    C. Only occurs in the postmenopausal woman.
    D. Diagnosis is made by careful history and physical examination.
    E. Lichen sclerosus presents as white premalignant lesions on the vulva.

55. **Menstruation:**
    A. Requires ovulation.
    B. Normally associated with 150 ml blood loss.
    C. Following ovulation, the corpus luteum secretes proges-
       terone.
    D. Anovulatory cycles are painless.
    E. Secretory phase is constant.

56. **Predisposing factors for primary postpartum haemorrhage
    include:**
    A. Twins.
    B. Postmaturity.
    C. Polyhydramnios.
    D. Previous scar on uterus.
    E. General anaesthesia with halothane.

57. **Acceptable methods to accelerate the first stage of labour
    include:**
    A. Rupture of membranes.
    B. Syntometrine.
    C. Prostin pessary.
    D. Oxytocin.
    E. Episiotomy.

58. **Bilateral salpingo-ophorectomy performed at the time of
    hysterectomy:**
    A. Performed for Stage I endometrial carcinoma.
    B. More technically difficult than hysterectomy with
       conservation of the ovaries.
    C. Requires oestrogen therapy in women < 40 years of age.
    D. Relieves premenstrual tension.
    E. Performed for Stage I carcinoma of the cervix.

59. **Causes of vulval ulcers include:**
    A. Squamous cell carcinoma.
    B. Primary syphilis.
    C. Behçet's disease.
    D. Lichen planus.
    E. *Herpes simplex.*

60. **Lactation:**
    A. Occurs 6 days after delivery.
    B. Oxytocin initiates milk production.
    C. Colostrum is produced on the first day postpartum.
    D. Engorgement occurs on the first day postpartum.
    E. Breast-feeding can be used as a natural method of
       contraception.

DRCOG MCQs for Circuit C
Questions

1. **Multiple pregnancy is associated with increased risk of:**
   A. Urinary tract infection.
   B. Cord prolapse.
   C. Antepartum haemorrhage.
   D. Anaemia.
   E. Polyhydramnios.

2. **Drugs that cross the placenta include:**
   A. Warfarin.
   B. Thyroxine.
   C. Iodine.
   D. Heparin.
   E. Carbimazole.

3. **Puerperal pyrexia may be due to:**
   A. Endometritis.
   B. Phlebitis.
   C. Breast abscess.
   D. Inverted uterus.
   E. Retained products of conception.

4. **Causes of preterm labour include:**
   A. Cone biopsy.
   B. Fetal malformation.
   C. Abruptio placenta.
   D. Pre-eclampsia.
   E. Multiple pregnancy.

5. **Complications of subtotal hysterectomy include:**
   A. Rectocoele.
   B. Anuria.
   C. Depression.
   D. Urinary tract infection.
   E. Vaginal vault prolapse.

6. **Bartholin's abscess:**
   A. Arises from the duct of the greater vestibular gland.
   B. May arise in an adenocarcinoma of the Bartholin's gland.
   C. Presents as an anterior swelling at the introitus.
   D. May contain *Escherichia coli*, *Staphylococcus* or gonococcal organisms.
   E. May be adequately treated by incision of the gland.

7. **Fetal causes of polyhydramnios include:**
   A. Oesophageal atresia.
   B. Anencephaly.
   C. Umbilical hernia.
   D. Spina bifida.
   E. Renal agenesis.

8. **Conditions predisposing towards breech presentation include:**
   A. Bicornuate uterus.
   B. Fibroid uterus.
   C. Spina bifida.
   D. Oligohydramnios.
   E. Placenta praevia.

9. **Indications for Caesarean section include:**
   A. Cephalopelvic disproportion.
   B. Placenta praevia.
   C. After vesicovaginal fistula repair.
   D. Transverse lie.
   E. Brow presentation.

10. **Predisposing factors towards intracranial haemorrhage in the newborn include:**
    A. Forceps delivery.
    B. Kernicterus.
    C. Birth asphyxia.
    D. Prematurity.
    E. Ventouse delivery.

11. **Local social services supply the following services:**
    A. Play schemes.
    B. Day nursery.
    C. Child-minding.
    D. Adoption centre.
    E. Nursery school.

12. **Adverse effects of the combined oral contraceptive (coc) pill include:**
    A. Increased risk of hepatocellular carcinoma.
    B. Hypertension.
    C. Relative risk of breast cancer of 1.24.
    D. Three-fold increase of myocardial infarction and ischaemic stroke in users with hypertension.
    E. Small increase in the relative risk of cervical cancer with a long duration of use.

27

13. **Combined oral contraceptive pill:**
    A. Consists of 21 days of ethinyloestradiol and progestogen and a 7-day pill-free period.
    B. Lowers the absolute risk of myocardial infarction.
    C. Lowers the risk of developing functional ovarian cysts.
    D. Lowers the risk of ovarian and endometrial cancer by 50% after 5 years of use.
    E. Treatment for both menorrhagia and dysmenorrhoea.

14. **Genital tract fistulae are associated with:**
    A. Hysterectomy.
    B. Forceps delivery.
    C. Endometriosis.
    D. Surgery for anterior vaginal wall prolapse.
    E. Surgery for urethral diverticula.

15. **Endometriosis may be associated with:**
    A. Deposits in lower abdominal scars.
    B. Chocolate cysts.
    C. Fixed retroverted uterus.
    D. Stricture formation in the bowel.
    E. Haemothorax.

16. **Pelvic endometriosis:**
    A. Diagnosed by transvaginal ultrasound.
    B. May present with deep dyspareunia, secondary dysmenorrhoea and ovulation pain.
    C. May be associated with infertility.
    D. May be associated with palpable tender nodules in the uterosacral ligament.
    E. Tends to regress at the menopause.

17. **Treatment for endometriosis may include:**
    A. Danazol.
    B. Norethisterone.
    C. Total hysterectomy with bilateral salpingo-oophorectomy.
    D. Diathermy.
    E. Local excision.

18. **Post-maturity is associated with:**
    A. Increased risk of perinatal mortality rate.
    B. Passage of meconium.
    C. 42/40 weeks' gestation and induction of labour is advisable.
    D. Meconium staining of the nails and cord.
    E. Placental insufficiency.

19. **Cardiac drugs that can be safely prescribed during pregnancy include:**
    A. Methyldopa.
    B. Atenolol.
    C. Hydralazine.
    D. Thiazides.
    E. Verapamil.

20. **Invasive cervical carcinoma is associated with:**
    A. HPV 16, 18 and 31.
    B. Sexual promiscuity.
    C. Smoking.
    D. Cervical intraepithelial neoplasia (CIN) III.
    E. Combined oral contraceptive pill.

21. **Ovarian tumours that secrete oestrogen include:**
    A. Arrhenoblastoma.
    B. Dysgerminoma.
    C. Teratoma.
    D. Granulosa cell tumour.
    E. Thecoma.

22. **Prematurity is associated with:**
    A. Increased risk of necrotizing enterocolitis.
    B. Hyaline membrane disease.
    C. Intraventricular haemorrhage.
    D. Persistent patent ductus arteriosus.
    E. Kernicterus.

23. **Endometrial hyperplasia is associated with:**
    A. Unopposed oestrogen stimulation.
    B. Dysfunctional uterine bleeding.
    C. Combined oral contraceptive pill.
    D. Hyperthyroidism.
    E. Granulosa-theca cell tumours.

24. **In pregnancy complicated by diabetes mellitus:**
    A. Insulin requirement rises during pregnancy.
    B. Insulin requirement increases immediately after delivery.
    C. Delivery should be arranged at 36 weeks to prevent late intrauterine death.
    D. Chlorpropamide may cause neonatal hypoglycaemia.
    E. Diabetes is confirmed by the 75 g oral glucose tolerance test.

25. **External cephalic version is contraindicated in:**
    A. Multiple pregnancy.
    B. Uterine scar.
    C. Antepartum haemorrhage.
    D. Rhesus-negative mother.
    E. 32 weeks' gestation.

26. **Pre-eclampsia is associated with:**
    A. Increased incidence in smokers.
    B. Increased perinatal mortality rate.
    C. Pregnancy > 20 weeks' gestation.
    D. Resolves within 10 days of delivery.
    E. Renal involvement may be detected early by monitoring uric acid levels.

27. **Investigations for pruritis vulvae include:**
    A. Urine for glycosuria.
    B. Endometrial curettage.
    C. Cervical smear.
    D. Vulval biopsy.
    E. High vaginal swab.

28. **Gynaecological operations:**
    A. Ventrosuspension is used to antevert the uterus.
    B. Manchester repair (Fothergill's operation) is used for a uterine prolapse.
    C. Wertheim's operation involves a total vaginectomy.
    D. Ovarian cystectomy is removal of the ovary containing the cyst.
    E. Transcervical ablation of the endometrium may result in pyometra.

29. **Features of uterine rupture include:**
    A. Vaginal bleeding.
    B. Violent uterine contractions.
    C. Intraperitoneal haemorrhage.
    D. Disappearance of the presenting part from the pelvis.
    E. Continuous postpartum haemorrhage (PPH) with a well-contracted uterus.

30. **Hyperemesis gravidarum may be associated with:**
    A. Liver failure.
    B. Pre-eclampsia toxaemia.
    C. Twin pregnancy.
    D. Hydatidiform mole.
    E. Polyneuritis.

31. **Features of the climacteric phase include:**
    A. Dyspareunia.
    B. Hot flushes.
    C. Scanty regular menstruation.
    D. Rise in follicle-stimulating hormone (FSH) during the first 7 days of the cycle.
    E. Poor memory and concentration.

32. **Hormone-replacement therapy (HRT):**
    A. May be administered intranasally.
    B. Owing to the first-pass effect through the liver, which requires lower doses of oral oestrogen to be administered than by the transdermal route.
    C. Standard dose of subcutaneously administered oestrogen is 50 mg and is effective for 6 months.
    D. Varicose veins are a relative contraindication for HRT.
    E. Otosclerosis is an absolute contraindication for HRT.

33. **Risk factors for osteoporosis include:**
    A. Chronic liver disease.
    B. Diabetes.
    C. Premature menopause.
    D. Cigarette smoking.
    E. Steroid therapy.

34. **Features of pre-eclampsia include:**
    A. Raised BP that develops after 16 weeks' gestation.
    B. Blurred vision.
    C. Epigastric pain.
    D. Hyper-reflexia.
    E. Spontaneous bleeding.

35. **Management of the newborn includes:**
    A. Performing the Guthrie test on the sixth day to detect raised levels of phenylalanine.
    B. Checking the umbilical stump for the presence of two veins and one artery and that separation has occurred by day 10.
    C. Regular BM stix for infants of diabetic mothers, as these infants are at particular risk of hyperglycaemia.
    D. Check that the respiratory rate is >60 breaths per minute.
    E. Administration of 1 mg vitamin K at birth to prevent haemorrhagic disease of the newborn.

36. **Appropriate investigations for recurrent miscarriages (RM) include:**
    A. Chromosomal karyotyping of both parents.
    B. Screening for antiphospholipid antibody and lupus anti-coagulant.
    C. Transvaginal ultrasound.
    D. Measure serum follicle-stimulating hormone (FSH) and luteinizing hormone (LH) in the mother.
    E. Hysterosalpingogram.

37. **Management of menorrhagia may include:**
    A. Norethisterone tablets 5 mg o tds for 10 days.
    B. Tranexamic acid 1 g o tds for 3 days.
    C. Placement on the combined oral contraceptive (coc) pill.
    D. Insertion of the Mirena intrauterine system.
    E. Mefenamic acid 500 mg o tds.

38. **Immunochemical urine pregnancy tests:**
    A. Unreliable after 19 weeks' gestation.
    B. Less precise than radioimmunoassay of β-hCG (human chorionic gonadotrophin).
    C. Should give a positive result 14 days after ovulation.
    D. Do not differentiate between hCG and luteinizing hormone (LH) and consequently may result in a false-positive pregnancy test.
    E. Depend on the detection of hCG produced by the conceptus.

39. *Chlamydia trachomatis:*
    A. Treated with oral erythromycin during pregnancy.
    B. Diagnosed on an endocervical swab.
    C. Chlamydial antigen and DNA may be detectable up to 3 weeks post-treatment.
    D. Most affected women are symptomless.
    E. Transmission risk during delivery may be as high as 70%.

40. **Mortality rates:**
    A. Maternal mortality rates are reported every 3 years.
    B. Maternal mortality rate is the number of maternal deaths while pregnant or within 42 days of abortion or delivery, not from accidental or incidental causes, per 100 000 births.
    C. Stillbirth mortality rate is the number of stillbirths after 24 weeks' gestation per 1000 total births.
    D. Neonatal mortality rate is the number of deaths of all live-born infants within the first 28 days per 1000 live births.
    E. Perinatal mortality rate is the number of stillbirths and first-week neonatal deaths per 1000 total births.

41. **Causes of pruritus vulvae include:**
    A. Crohn's disease.
    B. Iron deficiency anaemia.
    C. Lichen sclerosus.
    D. Lichen planus.
    E. Polycythaemia.

42. **Causes of dyspareunia include:**
    A. Fixed, retroverted uterus.
    B. Atrophic vaginitis.
    C. Postpartum perineal repair.
    D. Climacteric.
    E. Pelvic congestion.

43. **Characteristic features of ectopic pregnancy include:**
    A. Shoulder tip pain.
    B. Per vagina (PV) spotting.
    C. Amenorrhoea for < 10 weeks.
    D. Serum β-hCG > 6000 IU l^{-1}.
    E. 'Prune juice' blood loss as the decidua is lost from the uterus.

44. **Procidentia:**
    A. May cause postmenopausal bleeding.
    B. Because of atrophy of the cardinal and uterosacral ligaments.
    C. Second-degree uterine prolapse protruding from the introitus.
    D. May result from childbirth.
    E. May cause constipation.

45. **Management of procidentia may include:**
    A. Vaginal hysterectomy.
    B. Ring pessary.
    C. Topical oestrogen creams and packs if postmenopausal.
    D. Burch colposuspension.
    E. Fothergill's (Manchester) repair.

46. **Which maternal infections cause congenital defects to the fetus?**
    A. Poliomyelitis.
    B. Syphilis.
    C. *Listeria*.
    D. Cytomegalovirus.
    E. Toxoplasma.

47. **Maternal rubella:**
    A. May result in fetal patent ductus arteriosus.
    B. Diagnosed by chorionic villus sampling (CVS) after 8 weeks' gestation.
    C. If seronegative, the mother should be vaccinated in the puerperium.
    D. Recent infection is indicated by a positive rubella-specific IgM test.
    E. RNA virus; contracted though droplet infection.

48. **Ovarian carcinoma:**
    A. Stage III is defined as growth involving one or both ovaries with widespread intraperitoneal metastases.
    B. Combined oral contraceptive pill is protective.
    C. Spreads haematogenously.
    D. Has a higher mortality rate than cervical cancer due to its late presentation.
    E. In the management of ovarian carcinoma, surgery is generally followed by chemotherapy.

49. **Dysfunctional uterine bleeding:**
    A. Common at the extremes of reproductive life.
    B. Can be caused by carcinoma of the endometrium.
    C. Diagnosis of exclusion after organic pathology has been ruled out.
    D. Associated with a low follicle-stimulating hormone (FSH) level.
    E. May be treated by laser ablation of the endometrium.

50. **Compared with breast milk, cow's milk:**
    A. Contains more total protein content.
    B. Contains a higher concentration of calcium.
    C. Has a higher calorific value.
    D. Diarrhoea may result from cow's milk allergy.
    E. Contains IgA.

51. **Post-natal mastitis:**
    A. Usually occurs during the first postpartum week.
    B. Responsive to penicillin.
    C. Breast-feeding should be avoided during antibiotic therapy.
    D. Caused by *Streptococcus*.
    E. May be caused by a cracked nipple.

52. **Factors predisposing to primary postpartum haemorrhage (PPH) include:**
    A. Fibroids.
    B. Uterine atony.
    C. Von Willebrand's disease.
    D. Prior history of PPH.
    E. Warfarin therapy.

53. **ABO incompatibility:**
    A. Associated with a negative direct Coomb's test on a cord blood sample.
    B. Associated with neonatal jaundice within the first 24 hours of life.
    C. Can be detected antenatally.
    D. Due to iso-immunization.
    E. Most commonly associated with mothers of blood group O with infants of blood group A or B.

54. **Antepartum haemorrhage:**
    A. Fetal in origin in 0.5% of cases.
    B. Concealed in one-third of cases of placental abruptio.
    C. Vaginal examination is contraindicated.
    D. After 20 weeks requires a Kleihauer test in a rhesus-negative mother.
    E. Associated with raised maternal serum α-fetoprotein levels.

55. **46XX is associated with:**
    A. Hydatidiform mole.
    B. Turner's syndrome.
    C. Edward's syndrome.
    D. Sheehan's syndrome.
    E. Adrenogenital syndrome.

56. **Primary amenorrhoea is a feature of:**
    A. Granulosa-theca cell tumour.
    B. Turner's syndrome.
    C. Panhypopituitarism.
    D. Testicular feminization.
    E. Craniopharyngioma.

57. **Chorio-amnionitis:**
    A. May result in preterm labour.
    B. Necessitates intravenous broad-spectrum antibiotic therapy and induction of labour.
    C. Cannot occur if the fetal membranes are intact.
    D. Risk of infection increases with the duration of membrane rupture.
    E. May be caused by Group B *Streptococcus* infection ascending from the cervix.

58. **Raised maternal serum α-fetoprotein is characteristically found with:**
    A. Maternal liver disease.
    B. Hydatidiform mole.
    C. Intrauterine death.
    D. Multiple pregnancy.
    E. Exomphalos.

59. **Oligohydramnios is associated with:**
    A. < 200 ml liquor volume during the third trimester of pregnancy.
    B. Urethral aplasia.
    C. Prolonged pregnancy.
    D. Potter's syndrome.
    E. Talipes.

60. **Intrauterine growth restriction may be associated with:**
    A. Placental insufficiency.
    B. Oligohydramnios.
    C. Low socio-economic class.
    D. Raised maternal serum α-fetoprotein.
    E. Sickle cell disease.

DRCOG MCQs for Circuit A
Answers

1. **A C D**

This is a favourite DRCOG topic.

Guidelines for anti-D immunoglobulin suggest prophylaxis under the following sensitizing circumstances: spontaneous miscarriage after 12 weeks' gestation, spontaneous miscarriage with instrumentation (TOP), threatened miscarriage at any gestation, after falls or abdominal trauma. The dose of anti-D immunoglobulin is determined according to the level of exposure to rhesus-positive blood. Anti-D should be offered within 72 hours and covers the mother for the next 6 weeks. Anti-D prophylaxis is repeated at this time if bleeding persists. Routine antenatal prophylaxis according to the Royal College of Obstetricians and Gynaecologists for all rhesus-negative women consists of two doses of at least 500 IU anti-D immunoglobulin, the first dose at 28 weeks' gestation and the second dose at 34 weeks' gestation.

2. **B D**

This is a favourite DRCOG topic.

Risk factors for endometrial cancer include nulliparity, late menopause, diabetes, history of unopposed oestrogen administration, oestrogen-secreting tumours of the ovaries and obesity. Premarin is a form of unopposed oestrogen HRT and should only be administered to women post-hysterectomy.

3. **B C D E**

This is a favourite DRCOG topic.

Turner's syndrome is a gonadal dysgenesis syndrome associated with 45X0 karyotype in 50% of cases. There is a 10–20% chance of co-arctation of the aorta. The characteristics of Turner's include short stature (height rarely exceeding 1.5 m), short fourth metacarpals, lymphoedema of the hands and feet, webbing of the neck, and widely spaced nipples. The serum FSH level is high in infancy, falls initially during childhood but increases at 10 years of age. Serum LH levels rise and plasma oestradiol levels decrease.

4. **A C D**

This is a favourite DRCOG topic.

Routine blood tests offered at a booking clinic include full blood count, blood group and antibody screen, serology for hepatitis B (not A!), syphilis, rubella and HIV. Sickle cell test and haemoglobin electrophoresis are also offered to at-risk patients.

5. A

This is a favourite DRCOG topic.

Reversal of laparoscopic sterilization has been associated with a 25% success rate for open procedures and up to a 70% success rate with the aid of a microscope. Laparoscopic sterilization is not advisable at the time of Caesarean section, as it is associated with a higher failure rate. Laparoscopic sterilization has a small risk of postoperative ectopic pregnancy. As the procedure is done under general anaesthesia, a vasectomy under local anaesthesia poses less threat. Death from laparoscopic sterilization is 1 in 10 000 under a general anaesthesia versus 1 in 100 000 for a vasectomy performed under local anaesthesia. The failure rate for laparoscopic sterilization is 1 in 200 to 1 in 500.

6. A B E

This is a favourite DRCOG topic.

Increased levels of human chorionic gonadotrophin have been associated with choriocarcinoma, hyperemesis gravidarum, pregnancy and hydatidiform mole. Hepatoma may be associated with increased levels of α-fetoprotein. Ovarian cancer may be associated with elevated CA-125.

7. A D

Oligohydramnios may be associated with intrauterine growth retardation (IUGR), talipes, renal agenesis and pulmonary hypoplasia.

8. B C D E

Cervical smear may pick up incidental infections such as *Trichomonas vaginalis*, bacterial vaginosis (*Gardnerella*), actinomyces and *Candida*. A cervical smear may reveal mild-to-severe dysplasia, which is suggestive of low-to-high-grade cervical intraepithelial neoplasia (CIN). Severe dyskaryosis with additional features may suggest invasive carcinoma. Dyskaryotic glandular cells may represent adenocarcinoma of the endometrium or endocervical adenocarcinoma *in situ*.

9. A B C

This is a favourite DRCOG topic.

The Mirena coil or the levonorgestrel-releasing intrauterine system (IUS) is licensed to be used for 5 years at a time in the UK. It does not have a product licence yet for control of menorrhagia, but it does have this added advantage. The local effect of the Mirena coil causes thickening of the cervical mucus, endometrial atrophy and partial ovulation suppression. It is not advisable in patients with a history of PID and does not increase the risk of ectopic pregnancy. By acting as a contraceptive device with 99% efficacy, the risk is lower.

10. A D E

Puberty starts with the development of the breast bud at a median age of 9.8 years. The onset of pubic hair growth occurs at a median age of 10.5 years. Menarche usually occurs with further breast and areola enlargement at a median age of 12.8 years. Puberty may be associated with a cervical ectropion as may use of the oral contraceptive pill and pregnancy. Puberty may also be associated with dysfunctional uterine bleeding.

11. A B C D

This is a favourite DRCOG topic.

Post-coital bleeding is associated with cervical polyp, cervical ectropion, carcinoma of the cervix, infection with *Trichomonas vaginalis*, which may appear as a strawberry cervix, and atrophic vaginitis.

12. A E

This is a favourite DRCOG topic.

Deep dyspareunia is associated with PID, endometriosis, ectopic pregnancy, ovarian neoplasm and chronic pelvic pain. Superficial dyspareunia is associated with vulvar, vaginal or urethral pathology.

13. A B C D E

Intermenstrual bleeding may be associated with infection in patients with an IUD *in situ*.

14. A B C D E

This is a favourite DRCOG topic and may appear in MCQ or OSCE format!

The Pearl Index is expressed in terms of rate per 100 woman-years (HWY) and is calculated as follows:

Failure rate per HWY = total number of pregnancies × 1200/total months of use for all those using method.

Know how to calculate the index and the indices for all the forms of contraception.

15. A B C D E

This is a favourite DRCOG topic.

According to the *British National Formulary* (*BNF*), syntometrine is offered as routine management of the third stage of labour and is contraindicated during the first and second stages of labour. It can also be used to control bleeding due to incomplete abortion. Reported side-effects include nausea, vomiting, headache, dizziness, tinnitus, chest pain, palpitations, abdominal pain, dyspnoea, transient hypertension, stroke, myocardial infarction and pulmonary oedema.

When answering questions about drugs (indications, doses, contraindications, side-effects), be aware that the DRCOG examining panel relies on the *BNF* guidelines.

16. A C E

This is a favourite DRCOG topic.

Dr Apgar devised the Apgar scoring system in 1953. The newborn baby is assessed using five parameters taken at 1 and 5 minutes after birth. Scores range from 0 to 2 for each parameter. The Apgar score assesses heart rate (absent, < 100 or > 100 bpm), respiratory effort and **not** rate (absent, shallow/irregular or regular/crying), colour (pale/blue, body pink/extremities blue or pink), muscle tone (limp, some flexion or active flexion), and reflex irritability (none, grimace or cough/cry). A baby with a heart rate of < 100 bpm (1), with shallow respirations (not going by respiratory rate) (1), grimacing (1), with active flexion (not just moving all four limbs freely) (2) with blue extremities (1) would receive a total Apgar score = 6. Facemask resuscitation is indicated for a baby with no respiration and a heart rate < 100 bpm or one with irregular respirations and a heart rate > 100 bpm who fails to respond to gentle stimulation and opening and clearing the airway.

17. A B C D E

The differential diagnosis in this situation includes endometritis, retained products of conception, haematoma and breakdown of sutures. All options for investigation are appropriate for this patient.

18. A B C D E

Other causes for preterm labour include procedures such as amniocentesis, multiple pregnancy and an abnormal uterus.

19. A C D E

Hypothyroidism and not hyperthyroidism has been associated with pruritus vulvae. Other systemic causes include liver disease, skin diseases, polycythaemia and chronic renal failure. Local causes include scabies, pediculosis pubis, threadworms, candidiasis, atrophic vulvitis, vulval dystrophies and tumours.

20. A B C D E

Other potential complications of pre-eclampsia include fits, disseminated intracellular coagulopathy (DIC) and maternal death.

21. A B D E

Other neonatal risks in a mother with IDDM include a macrosomic baby, hypertrophic cardiomyopathy, severe hypoglycaemia, hypo-magnesaemia and not hypermagnesaemia, and increased risk of congenital anomaly. Congenital anomalies include anencephaly, meninogomyelocoele and sacral agenesis.

22. A B D

Obstetric risks to a pregnant woman with IDDM include pre-eclampsia, preterm labour, polyhydramnios and not oligo-hydramnios, and recurrent miscarriage.

23. A B C D E

Maternal causes of intrauterine growth retardation (IUGR) include smoking and alcohol, infections, pre-eclampsia or hyper-tension, placental abruption, diabetes mellitus, and renal disease. Fetal causes of IUGR include chromosomal abnormalities, anencephaly and multiple pregnancy.

24. A B C D E

Causes of symmetrical intrauterine growth retardation (IUGR) include TORCH (toxoplasmosis, rubella, cytomegalovirus and *Herpes simplex* viral infections) and chromosomal abnormalities such as Down's syndrome.

25. A B C D E

The signs and symptoms of PCO can include amenorrhoea or oligomenorrhoea, infertility, hirsutism, acne, obesity and bulimia. Management is based on whether the patient has plans for conceiving in the near future. If not, cyproterone acetate in the form of a combined oral contraceptive (coc) pill such as Dianette can be prescribed to combat acne and hirsutism. Otherwise, three courses of clomiphene citrate, ovulation induction or wedge resection of the ovaries can be suggested if the patient would like to conceive soon. A progesterone challenge test is advised for oligo- or amenorrhoea, and diet and psychotherapy for obesity and bulimia.

26. A B C D E

This is a favourite DRCOG topic.

According to the *British National Formulary* (BNF), the side-effects of clomiphene include visual disturbances, ovarian hyper-stimulation, hot flushes, abdominal discomfort, depression, insomnia, breast tenderness, headache, intermenstrual spotting, menorrhagia, endometriosis, convulsions, weight gain, rash and dizziness.

27. A D E

Causes of neonatal jaundice within the first 24 hours of life should be taken seriously and include excessive red cell haemolysis from rhesus or ABO incompatibility, congenital infection with toxo-plasmosis, rubella, cytomegalovirus, *Herpes* or hepatitis, glucose 6-phosphate dehydrogenase deficiency, Crigler–Najjar syndrome, hereditary spherocytosis, and increased red cell breakdown from polycythaemia or cephalhaematoma.

28. A B C D E

Causes of prolonged neonatal jaundice include congenital or acute infections, metabolic disease such as galactosaemia, endocrino-pathies such as hypothyroidism or hypopituitarism, α-1-antitrypsin deficiency, cystic fibrosis, intrahepatic biliary hypoplasia, intestinal obstruction and neonatal hepatitis.

29. A B C D E

Contraindications to oestrogen replacement therapy include un-diagnosed vaginal bleeding, acute and chronic liver disease, acute vascular thrombosis, migrainous headaches, endometrial and breast cancer.

30. A B C

Causes of dysmenorrhoea include endometriosis, misplaced IUD, pelvic inflammatory disease, ovarian tumour, history of sexual abuse, and prior abdominal or pelvic surgery. Fibroids are associated with menorrhagia. PCO is associated with amenorrhoea.

31. B C D E

This is a favourite DRCOG topic.

Malignant vulval carcinoma most commonly occurs in the 65–70-year age group. Risk factors include vulval irritation, obesity and HPV. Any stage other than Stage I is treated with radical vulvectomy and bilateral groin node dissection. Pelvic nodes that may become involved include the external iliac, femoral and superficial groin nodes.

32. A B C E

This is a favourite DRCOG topic.

Stage Ia cervical carcinoma is defined as carcinoma confined to the cervix, micro-invasive with a depth of invasion of < 3 mm into the stroma. It is diagnosed and may be treated by cone biopsy as long as there is no lymphatic involvement. Invasive carcinoma may be asymptomatic.

33. A B C D

This is a favourite DRCOG topic.

Meconium staining of the liquor is associated with fetal hypoxia, which may be caused by umbilical cord compression or uterine hypertonicity. Meconium staining is also associated with a post-term infant.

34. A B C D E

Human papilloma virus (HPV) is associated with all of the branches. HPV may be diagnosed on a cervical smear by the presence of koilocytes. HPV 16, 18 and 33 have been associated with cervical neoplasia. External genital warts may be treated with podophyllum paint (podophyllum resin 15% in compound benzoin tincture), condylline or warticon. However, podophyllum is contraindicated in pregnancy, as it is teratogenic. Flat warts on the cervix may be treated with cryotherapy.

35. A B C D

This is a favourite DRCOG topic.

The IUCD increases the relative risk of pregnancy. It is contraindicated in Wilson's disease (autosomal-recessive abnormality in the hepatic excretion of copper) and for patients with a copper allergy. It is also contraindicated for patients with PID, congenital or rheumatic heart disease, with fibroids or genital malignancy. It is replaced every 5 years. Menorrhagia or irregular bleeding is a relative contraindication to the IUCD. However, the IUS has been associated with controlling menorrhagia.

36. A B D E

This is a favourite DRCOG topic.

Bartholin's abscess may be due to *Gonococcus*, *Escherichia coli*, *Staphylococcus*, *Streptococcus* or anaerobic infection. The glands are also called the greater vestibular glands. Treatment for Bartholin's cyst and abscess is marsupialization, otherwise recurrence rate is high.

37. A B C D E

This is a favourite DRCOG topic.

The causes of vulval ulcers include Behçet's disease, chancroid caused by *Haemophilus ducreyi*, lymphogranuloma inguinale caused by *Chlamydia trachomatis*, granuloma inguinale caused by *Donovania granulomatis*, *Herpes simplex*, noma and tuberculosis.

38. A B E

This is a favourite DRCOG topic.

An ectopic pregnancy is one that occurs outside the uterine cavity. The majority occur in the Fallopian tube. Isthmial pregnancies may rupture between 4 and 8 weeks as the wall of the medial two-thirds of the tube cannot stretch. Ampullary pregnancies may rupture between 8 and 12 weeks as the muscle wall of the lateral one-third of the tube is lax. It occurs in 1 in 200 pregnancies and is associated with salpingitis, tubal surgery, IUD, etc. It may present with shoulder tip pain due to diaphragmatic irritation from accumulated blood. The abdominal pain may be bilateral or unilateral. Classically, the patient will have sudden, severe lower quadrant abdominal pain, a rigid abdomen, a very tender uterus and a boggy adnexal mass.

39. A C D E

This is a favourite DRCOG topic.

Clear cell and endometrioid tumours are almost all malignant. Dysgerminoma and immature teratoma are the most common malignant ovarian germ-cell tumours. Thirty per cent of serous, 15% of mucinous and < 5% of Brenner tumours are malignant. Three to 5% of Sertoli–Leydig cell tumours (arrhenoblastomas) are malignant. The Krukenberg tumour is a metastatic tumour from the stomach that contains signet-ring cells in the ovarian stroma.

40. A B D

This is a favourite DRCOG topic.

Trichomonas vaginalis and bacterial vaginosis (*Gardnerella*) cause offensive vaginal discharge. The latter is associated with a fishy odour and frequent vaginal douching or bubble baths. *Chlamydia* can produce an off-white vaginal discharge.

41. A B C D

The combined oral contraceptive (coc) pill contains oestrogen, which is absorbed in breast milk and, therefore, should not be offered as postpartum contraception.

42. A C D E

The maternal death rate per 1000 ectopic pregnancies for the UK from 1994 to 1996 was only 0.4. The causes of direct maternal deaths include thrombosis and thromboembolism, hypertensive disease of pregnancy, haemorrhage, amniotic fluid embolism, early pregnancy deaths (ectopics, spontaneous miscarriages, legal terminations), sepsis, genital tract trauma and anaesthetic complications.

43. A B C D E

This is a favourite DRCOG topic.

Tuberculous salpingitis often results in female sterility. Tuberculosis may also affect the male genital tract (prostate, seminal vesicles, epididymis) and present as non-tender nodular induration. Diagnosis may be made by endometrial biopsy showing tuberculous granulomas associated with a positive acid-fast bacilli culture. Diagnosis may also be made by an intradermal tuberculin skin test followed by a chest X-ray if the skin test is positive. According to the *British National Formulary* (*BNF*), the standard regimen for antituberculosis chemotherapy (isoniazid, rifampicin, pyrazinamide, ethambutol) may be given during pregnancy and breast-feeding. However, streptomycin is not advised during pregnancy.

44. A B C

This is a favourite DRCOG topic.

A uterus large for dates may be associated with twin pregnancy, gestational diabetes mellitus and a molar pregnancy. A 35-day menstrual cycle would result in an overestimation of the gestation by 1 week and would result in an estimated fundal height of less than expected for dates. Multiparity has no effect on the size of the fetus or uterus during pregnancy.

45. A B C D E

This is a favourite DRCOG topic.

Uterine retroversion is found in 20% of women. During pregnancy, a retroverted uterus corrects its position by 12–14 weeks and grows out of the bony pelvis. However, the retroverted uterus may become tethered in the Pouch of Douglas and result in anterior sacculation. This may then lead to dystocia in labour. If the retroverted uterus becomes tethered in the bony pelvis, growth is hindered, and the bladder displaces upwards into the abdomen. Retention of urine results from stretching of the urethra from bladder displacement. Management involves bed rest (lying prostrate) and an indwelling catheter and drainage. The uterus usually corrects itself.

46. B C D E

HIV is transmitted through blood, semen, breast milk and saliva.

47. A B D

Congenital hip dislocation should be detected at birth. There may be a family history of congenital dislocation or the baby may have been a breech presentation. Congenital hip dislocation is more common in females than in males. It is not a painful condition. The two tests for congenital hip dislocation are Ortolani's and Barlow's. Barlow's test is performed by placing the thumb into the baby's groin, grasping the upper thigh and levering the femoral head in and out of the acetabulum during abduction and adduction.

48. A B C D E

This is a favourite DRCOG topic.

Moniliasis or candidiasis may be associated with diabetes mellitus, pregnancy, immunosuppressive therapy, prolonged antibiotic use and steroid therapy.

49. A B C D E

Salpingitis is associated with sterility, ectopic pregnancy, tuberculosis, gonococcal infection and retrograde infection.

50. B C D E

A hydatidiform mole usually presents with vomiting and PV bleed during the first trimester or early second trimester. Vomiting in late pregnancy may be associated with a hiatus hernia, oesophageal reflux, pre-eclampsia, appendicitis and pyelopnephritis.

51. A C D E

This is a favourite DRCOG topic.

The differential diagnosis for postmenopausal bleeding includes carcinoma of the cervix and endometrium, endometrial polyp, and atrophic vaginitis. A speculum examination of the cervix and cervical smear are indicated. An urgent transvaginal ultrasound should be arranged to assess for endometrial hyperplasia or the presence of a polyp. A pipelle biopsy of the endometrium can then be taken if the endometrium is thickened.

52. A B C D E

Causes of proteinuria in pregnancy include acute pyelonephritis, urinary tract infection, pre-eclampsia, abruptio placenta, chronic glomerulonephritis, diabetic nephropathy and uncomplicated essential hypertension.

53. B E

This is a favourite DRCOG topic.

Endometrial hyperplasia is associated with polycystic sclerotic ovaries, oestrogen-producing tumours and unopposed oestrogen therapy. Endometrial hyperplasia is a risk factor for endometrial carcinoma and requires progestogen therapy either in the form of the combined oral contraceptive (coc) pill, the Mirena coil or HRT with progestogen, i.e. Prempak-C, in any woman with a uterus receiving oestrogen therapy.

54. A B C D E

Diabetes mellitus in pregnancy is associated with congenital anomalies (sacral agenesis, cardiac abnormalities), respiratory distress syndrome (RDS), intrauterine growth retardation (IUGR), prematurity, macrosomia, pre-eclampsia, preterm labour and polyhydramnios.

55. A C D E

The external cephalic version (ECV) is used to convert a breech presentation to a cephalic presentation. It is offered after 33 weeks. If the mother is rhesus-negative, anti-D immunoglobulin should be administered. Contraindications to performing ECV include antepartum haemorrhage, hypertension in the mother, multiple pregnancy, planned Caesarean delivery, a previous uterine scar from a Caesarean section and ruptured membranes.

56. A B D E

A breech presentation is associated with bony pelvic abnormalities, uterine anomalies, multiparity, prematurity, multiple pregnancy, placenta praevia and hydramnios. An abnormal lie is a contra-indication for forceps delivery. A footling or flexed breech presentation should be delivered by Caesarean section. A trial of vaginal delivery using Pinard's and Lovset's manoeuvre may be attempted for breech babies or the external cephalic version after 33 weeks.

57. A C

According to the *British National Formulary* (*BNF*), streptomycin is an aminoglycoside with the greatest potential for auditory and vestibular nerve damage and is contraindicated in pregnancy. Tetracycline has been shown to affect skeletal development in animal studies, causes dental discoloration and maternal hepato-toxicity with large parenteral doses. Trimethoprim is a folate antagonist and has theoretical teratogenic risk.

58. B C E

This is a favourite DRCOG topic.

Endometrial carcinoma is associated with obesity, diabetes, nulliparity, late menopause, prolonged menopause with excessive bleeding, oestrogen-secreting tumours of the ovaries (feminizing mesenchymoma), polycystic ovarian disease (sufferers tend to be obese), previous anovulatory cycles, unopposed oestrogen and dysfunctional uterine bleeding. HPV 16 and 18 are associated with cervical carcinoma.

59. A B C D

Chronic PID can present with symptoms of menorrhagia, congested dysmenorrhoea, pelvic pain, persistent mucopurulent vaginal discharge and sterility. Menorrhagia is associated with hypothyroidism and not hyperthyroidism. The causes of menorrhagia are legion and include adenomyosis (internal endometriosis), anticoagulation therapy, bicornuate uterus, blood dyscrasias, endometrial polyps, fibroids, IUD, hormonal and physiological factors.

60. A C D E

This is a favourite DRCOG topic.

Causes of PPH include DIC, hypofibrinogenaemia after abruptio placentae, placenta praevia, polyhydramnios, twins, previous scar on uterus and prolonged labour.

DRCOG MCQs for Circuit B
Answers

1. B C D E

Chlamydia trachomatis is a small Gram-negative obligate intracellular bacterium. In men, it is associated with non-gonococcal urethritis, epididymitis, proctitis, conjunctivitis and Reiter's syndrome. In women, it is associated with acute urethral syndrome, Bartholinitis, cervicitis, endometritis, salpingitis, conjunctivitis, perihepatitis (Fitz–Hugh–Curtis syndrome) and Reiter's syndrome. In the newborn, it can cause neonatal *Chlamydia* conjunctivitis and blindness. It is treated with oral doxycycline 100 mg bd for 7–14 days.

2. A B C D E

This is a favourite DRCOG topic.

Neisseria gonorrhoea is a Gram-negative diplococcus bacterium. In men, it causes urethritis, epididymitis, proctitis, conjunctivitis and pharyngitis (fellatio). In women, it causes acute urethral syndrome, bartholinitis, cervicitis, endometritis, salpingitis, conjunctivitis and perihepatitis. In the newborn, it is associated with gonococcal ophthalmia. According to the *British National Formulary* (*BNF*), treatment for gonorrhoea infection of the genital tract is ciprofloxacin or amoxycillin and probenecid.

3. A B C D E

Causes of transverse lie include contracted pelvis, fibroids, placenta praevia, polyhydramnios, relaxed uterus in grand multiparity, second twin and subseptate or arcuate uterus.

4. A B C D E

Causes of prolonged labour include relative cephalopelvic disproportion, inefficient uterine action, persistent occipitoposterior position, brow presentation and fetal hydrocephalus.

5. A B D E

Secondary dysmenorrhoea is defined as painful periods where an organic or psychosexual cause can be found. Causes include endometriosis, chronic PID, misplaced IUD and a history of sexual abuse.

6. B C E

Causes of neonatal jaundice within the first 24 hours of life include causes of excessive haemolysis (ABO or rhesus incompatibility), infection and increased red cell breakdown (cephalhaematoma, polycythaemia or bruising). This results in unconjugated hyperbilirubinaemia.

7. A B C D E

This is a favourite DRCOG topic.

Anovulatory cycles are associated with irregular bleeding and prolonged endometrial stimulation. This puts the woman at risk for endometrial hyperplasia and endometrial carcinoma.

8. A B C D E

Endometriosis can be found outside the uterus (in the intestine, in a surgical abdominal scar, etc.) or within the myometrium (adenomyosis). It presents with secondary dysmenorrhoea, deep dyspareunia and ovulatory pain.

9. A B D

Vesicovaginal fistula is associated with recurrent UTIs and continuous wetting, and it may be caused by carcinoma of the cervix.

10. A C E

Secondary amenorrhoea is associated with hypotholamic amenorrhoea (anorexia nervosa), premature menopause, polycystic ovarian disease, myxoedema and thyrotoxicosis.

11. D E

This is a favourite DRCOG topic.

Cryptomenorrhoea is defined as retention of menstrual blood. It occurs due to anatomical obstruction of menstrual flow. The most common cause is an imperforate hymen. Atresia of the Müllerian ducts may lead to cryptomenorrhoea and haematocolpus. Chromosomal abnormality and absence of secondary sexual characteristics suggest primary amenorrhoea. Short stature suggests Turner's syndrome (gonadal dysgenesis) and primary amenorrhoea.

12. A B C D E

This is a favourite DRCOG topic.

Sarcoma botyroides is a 'grape-like' mixed mesodermal tumour that occupies the vaginal vault and can present with PV bleeding. Urethral prolapse can become excoriated, raw and bleed. Granulosa thecal cell tumour and dysgerminoma are oestrogen-secreting tumours of the ovary and are associated with precocious pseudopuberty. Other causes of precocious pseudopuberty include adrenal tumours, hypothyroidism, McCune–Albright syndrome and oestrogen-containing medication.

13. A B C D E

This is a favourite DRCOG topic.

The success rates for open reversal of laparoscopic sterilization are only 25% versus the microscopic approach (70%). The early complication rate is < 5% and includes bleeding and infection. The late complication is pregnancy, which is likely to be ectopic. The morbidity rate associated with laparoscopic sterilization is higher than that associated with vasectomy performed under local anaesthesia. This latter option should be discussed when counselling a woman on sterilization.

14. A B

Adenomyosis is endometriosis within the myometrium and presents as secondary dysmenorrhoea.

15. A D

The factors that increase the success of vaginal delivery after Caesarean section include a normal vaginal delivery after the first Caesarean section and a non-recurrent indication for the previous Caesarean section. A previous lower segment approach for Caesarean section rather than a classical approach is amenable to trial of scar (TOS).

16. A B D E

This is a favourite DRCOG topic.

Postpartum DVT presents with low-grade pyrexia, unilateral lower leg oedema, calf tenderness, a positive Homan's sign (pain on dorsiflexion), and pain on palpation of the deep veins of the calf. Blood group O is said to be protective against DVTs. Risk factors for postpartum DVT include multiparity, increased maternal age, classical Caesarean section, immobility and a previous history of DVT.

17. All false

This is a favourite DRCOG topic.

Sodium valproate is associated with increased risk of neural tube defects, neonatal bleeding and neonatal hepatotoxicity. Propranolol or β-blockers are associated with intrauterine growth retardation (IUGR), neonatal hypoglycaemia and bradycardia. ACE inhibitors adversely affect fetal and neonatal blood pressure control and renal function and have been associated with skull defects and oligohydramnios. Carbamazepine is associated with increased risk of neural tube defects and neonatal bleeding. NSAIDs may cause closure of the fetal ductus arteriosus *in utero* and persistent pulmonary hypertension of the newborn.

18. A B C D E

Anencephaly has an incidence of 1 in 5000 births. It is more common in girls and associated with polyhydramnios. Diagnosis is made on ultrasound and abdominal palpation. Plasma and amniotic fluid α-fetoprotein levels are raised. Shoulder dystocia and death on delivery are to be expected.

19. A B C

Recognized sequelae of salpingitis include chronic pelvic pain, ectopic pregnancy, infertility and tubo-ovarian abscess.

20. B C D E

Post-coital bleeding may be caused by atrophic vaginitis, cervical ectropion, cervical carcinoma or cervical polyp. Cervical ectropion is eversion of the lower cervical canal and is associated with the three 'p's': puberty, pregnancy and the combined oral contraceptive (coc) pill. It is usually asymptomatic but can present with post-coital bleeding. Treatment involves cryotherapy.

21. B C D E

Caesarean section delivery is advised if the mother's viral load is high and the CD4 count low. Vaginal delivery is possible if the viral load is low and the CD4 count is negative. According to the *British National Formulary* (BNF) guidelines, Zidovudine or AZT is administered to the infant from the first 12 hours of life to at least 6 weeks of age. AZT is also administered to the mother from 14 weeks' gestation to labour and then by intravenous therapy until the umbilical cord is clamped.

22. A B C D E

This is a favourite DRCOG topic.

Complications of hysterectomy include haemorrhage, wound infection, wound haematoma, atelectasis, bronchopneumonia, urinary retention, urinary tract infection, injury to the ureter or bowels, uterovaginal fistula, vesicovaginal fistula, thrombophlebitis, deep vein thrombosis (DVT), pulmonary embolism and pelvic abscess.

23. B C D E

This is a favourite DRCOG topic.

Oestrogen limits the loss of bone mass. It does not increase bone mass. HRT in the postmenopausal woman must be taken for at least 5 years for the effects to be beneficial. Raloxifene is a selective oestrogen receptor modulator and has an oestrogen-like effect on bones and the vagina. It has an anti-oestrogen effect on the breasts and endometrium but does not diminish menopausal vasomotor symptoms. Osteoporosis is characterized by a decrease in cortical thickness and a decrease in the number and size of trabeculae of cancellous bone. Statistically, one in two women > 70 years of age will have an osteoporotic-related fracture, and one in four women in her 60's will have an osteoporotic-related fracture. Bisphosphonates such as etidronate are a recognized therapy for postmenopausal spinal osteoporosis.

24. A B C D E

Risk factors for osteoporosis include low body weight, lack of physical activity, family history of osteoporosis, smoking and excess alcohol intake.

25. A B C D E

This is a favourite DRCOG topic.

DIC is associated with abruptio placentae, severe pre-eclampsia or eclampsia, amniotic fluid embolism, sepsis, intrauterine fetal demise and transfusion reaction.

26. B C D E

This is a favourite DRCOG topic.

Hyperemesis gravidarum is more common with first pregnancies but can recur in subsequent pregnancies. Metoclopramide or maxolon may be administered with intravenous fluid boluses of Hartmann's solution. Maxolon as well as the phenothiazines have been associated with acute dystonic reactions and oculogyric crises. Hyperemesis gravidarum may be associated with multiple pregnancies and a hydatidiform mole, which should be excluded by transvaginal ultrasound. If untreated, the condition may progress to hypovolaemia, electrolyte imbalance and death from liver failure.

27. A C D E

This is a favourite DRCOG topic.

Of Down's syndrome, 95% is of non-disjunctional events leading to 47 chromosomes with an extra number 21 autosome. A total of 4% and not 20% of Down's syndrome is due to translocation with 46 chromosomes and the extra number 21 attached to the autosome. Of Down's syndrome, 1% is mosaics. The overall incidence of Down's syndrome is 1 in 650 live births. The maternal age-related risk of Down's is ~1 in 365 at age 35 years and 1 in 110 at age 40 years. Down's syndrome is associated with mental deficiency, short stature, muscle hypotonia, hyperflexibility of the joints, brachycephaly, short neck, narrow palate, typical facies, gaps between the first and second toes, incurving fifth finger, transverse palmar creases, dermatoglyphics, congenital heart disease, duodenal atresia, Brushfield's spots of the iris, conjunctivitis, and a risk of developing leukaemia.

28. A B C D E

This is a favourite DRCOG topic.

The contraceptive diaphragm is 92–96% effective if used properly. Each woman must be fitted according to the distance between the posterior fornix and the symphysis pubis. The diaphragm should be used in conjunction with two strips of spermicide and left in place for at least 6 hours after intercourse has taken place but < 30 hours to avoid toxic shock syndrome. The diaphragm will need to be refitted if the woman loses or gains 3 kg in weight, delivers a baby, has a miscarriage or TOP.

29. A B C

This is a favourite DRCOG topic.

Face presentation may be associated with anecephaly, dolichocephaly (long head), lax uterus, multiple pregnancy or polyhydramnios. Maternal congenital hip dislocation may give rise to cephalopelvic disproportion. Fibroids are more associated with shoulder presentation by preventing the engagement of the head in the pelvis.

30. A C E

This is a favourite DRCOG topic.

Fibroids may present with anaemia from menorrhagia, dysmenorrhoea, urinary retention or intermenstrual bleeding.

31. A B C D E

This is a favourite DRCOG topic.

Asymptomatic bacteriuria occurs in ~5% of pregnant women and is defined as the asymptomatic presence of > 100 000 bacteria ml^{-1} urine. Asymptomatic bacteriuria is associated with an up to 30% risk of acute pyelonephritis and should be treated with amoxycillin for 5 days. The bacteria associated with asymptomatic bacteriuria include *Escherichia coli* and *Proteus mirabilis*. Asymptomatic bacteriuria is associated with preterm labour if left untreated.

32. A B C D

This is a favourite DRCOG topic.

Dyspareunia may be associated with the climacteric due to atrophy of the vagina and vulva with menopause, PID, endometriosis, malignant diseases of the uterus and ovaries, fixed retroversion of the uterus, inflammatory conditions of the vulva or vagina, etc.

33. A B C E

This is a favourite DRCOG topic.

The risk factors for respiratory distress syndrome (RDS) include a diabetic mother, small for gestational age (SGA) with a birth weight < 10% for gestation, prematurity, and a lecithin/sphingomyelin ratio < 2 and no phosphatidylglycerol. Steroid therapy is administered to prevent RDS in premature infants between 28 and 32 weeks' gestation.

34. A B C D E

All of the above conditions occur in pregnancy. The folic acid requirements for prevention of recurrence of neural tube defects are 5 mg folic acid daily until week 12 of pregnancy. Other changes occurring with pregnancy include an increase in cardiac output, a decrease in peripheral resistance, a decrease in systolic and diastolic blood pressure until the third trimester, and, possibly, a third heart sound or a systolic ejection murmur.

35. A B E

A newborn's heart rate should be > 100 and is evaluated at 1 and 5 minutes using the Apgar scoring system. Physiological jaundice occurs in 50% of newborns on days 2 or 3.

36. B C D E

Trichomonas vaginalis is a sexually transmitted disease and is readily diagnosed under the microscope in a drop of saline. *T. vaginalis* is a flagellated protozoon and may infect the vagina, cervix, urethra and Bartholin's glands. It causes a frothy yellow-green purulent vaginal discharge. It is amenable to a 5-day course of metronidazole therapy.

37. A C D

Cervical erosion or ectropion may be a cause of intermenstrual bleeding and can be treated by cryotherapy if symptomatic. It commonly occurs in pregnancy, in patients on the oral contraceptive pill or at birth. Columnar eversion of the endocervical glandular tissue may be asymptomatic. The diagnosis is confirmed by colposcopy.

38. A D

PIH or pre-eclampsia may occur with twin pregnancy and hydatidiform mole and is almost exclusively seen in first pregnancies.

39. A B C E

The indications for forceps delivery are failure of progress in the second stage, fetal distress or maternal compromise and to prevent fetal or maternal morbidity. Requirements for forceps delivery include engaged head, ruptured membranes, a fully dilated cervix, an empty bladder and rectum, epidural anaesthesia, and a known head position.

40. A B D E

This is a favourite DRCOG topic.

Endometrial carcinoma is more common in the postmenopausal woman with a median age of 60 years. This compares to a median age of 52 years for cervical carcinoma. Ovarian carcinoma is the most common genital tract tumour in England and Wales, followed by cervical carcinoma and then endometrial. Endometrial carcinoma is the most common genital tract tumour in the USA and parts of Australia. The majority of endometrial carcinoma is adenocarcinoma of the endometrium and not squamous cell carcinoma. Stages Ic and II are correctly listed according to the International Federation of Gynaecology and Obstetrics (FIGO).

41. A C E

The first stage of labour may be shortened by AROM, oxytocin or Caesarean section. Forceps only play a role in the second stage of labour.

42. D E

The treatment of PPH involves resuscitation of the patient, rubbing the uterus, intravenous ergometrine and not ergotamine, intravenous syntocinon drip, uterine exploration, and, if all else fails, laparotomy with internal iliac ligation or hysterectomy.

43. A B C D E

This is a favourite DRCOG topic.

Ectopic pregnancies are 97% tubal in location and most implant in the ampulla. Having one ectopic pregnancy is a risk factor for having a second. Blood loss may be dark like prune juice and represents the shedding of decidual endometrium. Presentation may include unilateral abdominal pain, amenorrhoea, PV bleed, adnexal mass or referred pain via the phrenic nerve to the shoulder tip secondary to diaphragmatic irritation.

44. B C D E

This is a favourite DRCOG topic.

Unstable lie may be associated with fetal abnormalities, uterine fibroids, placenta praevia, multiparity and fetal macrosomia. Unstable lie is not associated with congenital anomalies of the uterus.

45. A B C D E

This is a favourite DRCOG topic.

Puerperal psychosis is associated with 1 in 500 births and is characterized by suicidal tendencies, schizophrenic delusions, mania and/or severe depression. Hospitalization with the baby is mandatory for treatment with antidepressants and antipsychotics.

46. A B D

This is a favourite DRCOG topic.

Haemoglobin < 10 g dl^{-1} may be due to iron or folate deficiency. Oral iron supplementation takes months to correct iron deficiency anaemia. Megaloblastic anaemia and aplastic anaemia are known side-effects of anticonvulsant drugs.

47. A B D E

This is a favourite DRCOG topic.

The coexistence of varicose veins is not strongly associated with deep venous thrombosis.

48. A B

The treatment of PCO consists of the combined oral contraceptive pill to reduce bleeding, anti-androgen drugs such as cyproterone acetate (in Dianette, the oral contraceptive pill) and clomiphene to induce ovulation. Patients with PCO are at risk of ovarian hyperstimulation on clomid. Tranexamic acid and zoladex are used in the treatment of fibroids and not PCO. Danazol is used in the treatment of endometriosis.

49. A B C D E

This is a favourite DRCOG topic.

PCO may be associated with all of the above.

50. A B C D E

This is a favourite DRCOG topic.

Primary postpartum haemorrhage may be associated with amniotic fluid embolism, low placenta, polyhydramnios, placenta abruptio, prolonged labour, pulmonary embolism, retained placenta, trauma to the uterus or cervix, twins, uterine atony, uterine inversion, uterine malformation or fibroids.

51. D E

Endometrial carcinoma is diagnosed by Pipelle biopsy of the lining of the endometrial cavity. Bacterial vaginosis or *Gardnerella* is diagnosed by the visualization of clue cells on Gram stain of the high vaginal swab.

52. A B C

This is a favourite DRCOG topic.

Absolute contraindications to the use of the IUCD include known or suspected pregnancy, undiagnosed abnormal vaginal bleeding, suspected malignancy of the genital tract, recent STD or PID in the past 3 months, a distorted uterine cavity due to fibroids, and copper allergy or Wilson's disease. Relative contraindications to the use of the IUCD include menorrhagia and anaemia, multiple sex partners, young and nulliparous women, recent PID, valvular heart disease (risk of subacute bacterial endocarditis), recent benign trophoblastic disease, immunosuppressive therapy, and current anticoagulant therapy.

53. A C

Metropathia haemorrhagica (cystic hyperplasia) is more common in menopausal women.

54. A B

Vulvar dystrophies include hyperplastic dystrophy, lichen sclerosus, leukoplakia and VIN. The most common symptom is pruritus. The malignant potential is < 5%. Definitive diagnosis is made by biopsy of the lesion. Lichen sclerosus is due to elastic tissue turning to collagen with the vulva becoming white, flat and shiny. This is not premalignant. Treatment is with 3% testosterone cream. However, leukoplakia may be premalignant and presents as white patches on and around the vulva. Treatment is with topical corticosteroids.

55. C D

Menstruation does not always require ovulation and is normally associated with 50 ml blood loss. Oestrogen in the proliferative phase promotes endometrial proliferation. Following ovulation, progesterone is secreted by the corpus luteum. Glands become tortuous and the stroma oedematous. Spiral arteries extend to the superficial layers of the endometrium and become convoluted. If pregnancy does not occur by day 23, the corpus luteum regresses and the endometrium undergoes involution. Marked constriction of the spiral arterioles causes ischaemia of the endometrium and the resulting necrosis causes the sloughing of the endometrium.

56. A B C D E

This is a favourite DRCOG topic.

Predisposing factors for PPH include high parity, twins, prolonged labour, previous scar on the uterus, general anaesthesia with halothane, polyhydramnios, cervical tear, and the presence of fibroids.

57. A C D

The first stage of labour involves descent of the fetal head and cervical dilatation. Syntometrine is used to aid delivery of the placenta in the third stage of labour. An episiotomy is only performed in the second stage of labour.

58. A C E

For Stage I carcinoma of the cervix, a Wertheim's radical abdominal hysterectomy is advocated, which also includes removal of the broad ligaments, parametria, the upper two-thirds of the vagina and the regional lymph nodes.

59. A B C E

This is a favourite DRCOG topic.

The causes of vulval ulcers include Behçet's, primary syphilis (painless ulcer), chancroid, lymphogranuloma inguinale, granuloma inguinale, *Herpes simplex*, squamous cell carcinoma of the vulva and tuberculosis. Lichen planus is a cause of oral ulcers on the buccal mucosa.

60. C E

Colostrum is produced from day 1 or 2 and contains protein, fat, minerals and secretory IgA. Mature milk is produced from day 3. Engorgement takes place on day 3 postpartum. Human placental lactogen initiates milk production and suckling stimulates the release of prolactin and oxytocin. Oxytocin then causes contractions of the myoepithelial cells in the alveoli and milk ducts. Breast-feeding can be used as a natural form of contraception as long as the baby is < 6 months of age and is on full feeds with breast milk and if the mother is amenorrhoeic. The risk of pregnancy is then only 2%. Otherwise, the progestogen-only pill should be offered on day 21 after childbirth or the IUCD 5–6 weeks postpartum.

DRCOG MCQs for Circuit C
Answers

1. B C D E

Multiple pregnancy is associated with an increased risk of anaemia (folate and iron deficiencies), APH, polyhydramnios, malpresentation, cord prolapse and PPH.

2. A B C E

Only heparin can safely be administered during pregnancy.

3. A B C E

The causes of puerperal pyrexia include urinary tract infections, infections of the genital tract, breast infections and thromboembolic events.

4. A B C D E

The causes of preterm labour include amnionitis, APH, cervical incompetence, cone biopsy, diabetes, fetal abnormalities, multiple pregnancy, polyhydramnios, pre-eclampsia, pyelonephritis and uterine abnormalities.

5. A B C D E

This is a favourite DRCOG topic.

The complications of subtotal hysterectomy include bleeding, pelvic cellulitis, abscess or haematoma, injury to the ureter, bladder or intestines, ureterovaginal fistula, thrombophlebitis, pulmonary embolism, vaginal vault prolapse, urinary tract infection, or rectocoele.

6. A B D

This is a favourite DRCOG topic.

Bartholin's glands are paired greater vestibular glands in the posterior ends of the labia minora. An abscess may arise from a retention cyst, which becomes secondarily infected with *Escherichia coli*, *Staphylococcus* or gonococcal organisms. Treatment requires marsupialization.

7. A B C D

This is a favourite DRCOG topic.

Fetal causes of polyhydramnios include anencephaly (unable to swallow), spina bifida, umbilical hernia, oesophageal or duodenal atresia, ectopia vesicae and hydrops fetalis. Renal agenesis results in oligohydramnios.

8. A B C D E

Conditions predisposing towards breech presentation include bicornuate uterus, fibroid uterus, hydrocephalus, oligohydramnios, placenta praevia and spina bifida.

9. A B C D E

Indications for Caesarean section include CPD, some malpresentations such as transverse lie, brow presentation, breech presentation in multiple pregnancy, mentoposterior presentation, placenta praevia, after vaginal surgery, severe pre-eclampsia, abruptio placenta, fetal distress, prolapsed cord, failed induction, failure to progress and failed trial of scar.

10. A C D E

This is a favourite DRCOG topic.

Intracranial haemorrhage in the newborn is commonly associated with hypoxia and prematurity. It is also a rare complication of instrumental delivery. Kernicterus is associated with athetoid cerebral palsy and sensorineural deafness.

11. A B C D E

This is a favourite DRCOG topic.

According to the North District Social Services Department on Offley Road, London SW9, all of the choices are true.

12. A C D E

This is a favourite DRCOG topic.

According to the Faculty of Family Planning and Reproductive Health Care and the Royal College of Obstetricians and Gynaecologists, the adverse effects of the combined oral contraceptive (coc) pill include increased risk of breast and cervical cancer, and a three-fold increase in relative risk of myocardial infarction and ischaemic stroke for users with concomitant hypertension. For smokers, the relative risk of myocardial infarction is ten times higher and two times higher for ischaemic stroke.

13. A C D E

The use of the combined oral contraceptive (coc) pill does not lower the absolute risk of myocardial infarction. The absolute risk of myocardial infarction is very low in young women, and actually increases with smoking or hypertension.

14. A B D E

Endometriosis is associated with extrauterine endometrial deposits that may lead to obstruction (renal, bowel, etc.), adhesions, pelvic pain, etc. depending on the location of the deposits. Fistula formation is associated with vaginal or bladder surgery and obstetric complications.

15. A B C D E

The typical picture for endometriosis is a fixed, retroverted uterus (from adhesions between the ovaries and posterior uterus), enlarged, tender ovaries (containing blood-filled or chocolate endometrial cysts), and tender, palpable nodules in the uterosacral ligament. Foci of endometrium may be found in the lungs (haemothorax), umbilicus, lower abdominal scars, bladder (haematuria), bowel, peritoneum, ureters and vaginal wall.

16. B C D E

Endometriosis is best diagnosed by laparoscopy with biopsy. Endometriosis may be due to retrograde menstruation and tends to regress at menopause.

17. A B C D E

All the above are acceptable methods of treatment for endometriosis. Danazol inhibits pituitary gonadotrophin secretion and at 800 mg daily for 6 months suppresses menstruation. Androgenic side-effects include acne, hirsutism, voice deepening (irreversible) and weight gain. Norethisterone, at 10–15 mg daily starting on day 5 for 4–6 months, is also an acceptable progestogen form of therapy for suppression of menstruation. Side-effects include nausea, vomiting, weight gain and fluid retention. Surgical methods include diathermy or local excision of the endometriotic tissue or total hysterectomy and BSO.

18. A B C D E

This is a favourite DRCOG topic.

All are associated with post-maturity defined as gestation > 42 weeks. There is a two-fold increase in perinatal mortality rate (5/1000 to 10/1000). Problems encountered include oligohydramnios, passage of meconium, obstructed labour (from macrosomia), placental insufficiency (from ageing and infarction of the placenta) and fetal distress. Induction of labour is advisable after 42 weeks with a lower tolerance to perform a Caesarean section. Post-natal signs of post-maturity include dry, cracked and loose skin, long fingernails, meconium staining of nails, fetal membranes, skin and umbilical cord, and the loss of subcutaneous fat.

19. A C

Atenolol or β-blockers are associated with intrauterine growth retardation (IUGR), neonatal hypoglycaemia and bradycardia. Hydralazine is safe when administered in the third trimester. Verapamil or calcium-channel blockers may inhibit labour, but the risk is weighed against management of uncontrolled maternal hypertension. Thiazides are associated with neonatal thrombocytopaenia.

20. A B C D E

All are associated with cervical carcinoma. Severe dysplasia or carcinoma *in situ* is defined as cervical intraepithelial neoplasia (CIN) III and most progress to invasive cervical carcinoma by 10 years.

21. D E

Be aware that oestrogen-secreting ovarian tumours may give rise to endometrial hyperplasia and endometrial carcinoma. These tumours may also present with sexual pseudoprecocity in children. Arrhenoblastomas (Sertoli–Leydig cell tumours) are associated with masculinization and rarely with malignancy. Teratomas are the second most common malignant ovarian germ-cell tumour and contain neural elements, cartilage and epithelial tissue.

22. A B C D E

Prematurity or a baby born < 37 weeks gestation is at risk of developing all the conditions.

23. A B E

This is a favourite DRCOG topic.

Endometrial hyperplasia results from persistently high levels of oestrogen, unopposed by progesterone. Even HRT in the form of topical oestrogen vaginal creams should be used with caution as absorption can result in endometrial hyperplasia.

24. A D E

Diabetes is confirmed by the 75 g OGTT. Insulin requirements rise during pregnancy but fall during labour and immediately after delivery. Nowadays, delivery can be postponed closer to term with good antenatal care.

25. A B C E

External cephalic version is offered after 33 weeks to convert a breech presentation to cephalic.

26. B C D E

Pre-eclampsia is a condition associated with pregnancy at >20 weeks. Smokers have a decreased incidence of pre-eclampsia. Pre-eclampsia is associated with primiparity, positive family history, short stature, being underweight, pre-existing migraine, hypertension, renal disease, placental hydrops (rhesus disease), hydatidiform mole and multiple pregnancy. Proteinuria is a late sign of the disease. Monitoring of uric acid levels gives an earlier indication of renal involvement.

27. A C D E

Investigations for pruritus vulvae include cervical smear, vulval and vaginal swabs, testing for glycosuria, and vulval biopsy. Causes for pruritus vulvae include general (psoriasis, lichen planus) and local (infection, vaginal discharge, infestation or vulval dystrophy).

28. B D E

Wertheim's hysterectomy for cervical carcinoma includes removal of local lymph nodes and a cuff of vagina. Transcervical ablation of the endometrium by laser or diathermy may be used as an alternative to hysterectomy, but it is associated with pyometra as a complication. Scarring from opposed ablated surfaces results in adhesions at the cervical canal and resultant pyometra if a small focus of endometrial tissue is left behind. Treatment then involves a hysteroscopy and cervical dilatation to allow the 'hidden blood' to escape from the uterine cavity and prevent reoccurrence.

29. A C D E

Uterine rupture is not associated with violent uterine contractions but rather the cessation of contractions. Rupture may precede labour as in a Caesarean scar dehiscence, the most common cause for uterine rupture. Predisposing conditions to uterine rupture also include obstructed labour in the multiparous with concomitant use of oxytocin, high forceps delivery and breech extraction.

30. A B C D E

This is a favourite DRCOG topic.

All may manifest during pregnancy as hyperemesis gravidarum. Polyneuritis results from vitamin B deficiency.

31. A B C D E

The climacteric phase is the perimenopausal phase and is characterized by the increased resistance of the ovarian follicle to stimulation by the gonadotrophins. There is a rise in FSH during the first 7 days of the cycle. Scanty regular menstruation may occur for up to 3 years before menopause occurs. Menopause is defined as 12 months of amenorrhoea and is associated with FSH > 30 IU l^{-1}.

32. A C D

HRT may be administered by oral, subcutaneous, transdermal, intranasal, sublingual or vaginal routes. Owing to the first-pass effect through the liver, higher and not lower doses of oral oestrogen are required. Varicose veins are a relative contra-indication for HRT, as is hypertension, smoking, diabetes, gall-stones, migraines, fibroids, previous DVT, previous myocardial infarction, endometriosis and endometrial cancer. Otosclerosis is a relative contraindication. Absolute contraindications to HRT include active thromboembolic disease, breast cancer, pregnancy, severe, active liver disease and unexplained vaginal bleeding.

33. A B C D E

Risk factors for osteoporosis include Caucasian race, chronic liver disease, smoking, diabetes, immobilization, premature menopause, slight and small build, and steroid therapy.

34. B C D E

Pre-eclampsia is defined as hypertension associated with protein-uria that develops after 20 weeks gestation. It may be associated with epigastric pain, a tender liver (elevated LFTs), spontaneous bleeding and bruising (low platelet count), hyper-reflexia, blurred vision (signs of increased intracranial pressure) and oliguria (increased urate and proteinuria).

35. A E

The Guthrie or heel prick test is performed on day 6 to exclude phenylketonuria. The umbilical stump should contain two arteries and one vein and it usually separates between days 8 and 10. Infants of diabetic mothers are at risk of hypoglycaemia and not hyperglycaemia. The respiratory rate should be < 60 breaths per minute. If it is > 60, think respiratory distress syndrome (RDS).

36. A B C D E

This is a favourite DRCOG topic.

Investigations for recurrent miscarriages (RM) include full blood count, serum FSH and LH levels in the mother, chromosomal karyotyping of both parents, screening for antiphospholipid antibodies, anticardiolipin and lupus anticoagulant, high vaginal and endocervical swabs, and transvaginal ultrasound (to exclude anatomical anomaly). A hysterosalpingogram and hysteroscopy may also be indicated if the ultrasound is suggestive. Parental chromosome abnormality is found in 3–5% of couples. Antiphospholipid antibodies are found in 15% of women. Bacterial vaginosis and cervical incompetence are two causes of second trimester miscarriages.

37. A B C D E

All are recognized treatments for menorrhagia. If menorrhagia is secondary to fibroids, a transvaginal ultrasound should be arranged to exclude distortion of the endometrial cavity by fibroids before insertion of an IUS.

38. A B C E

The sensitivity of a urine pregnancy test is set high enough to detect 500 or 1000 IU hCG l^{-1} urine so that the detection of LH cannot result in a false-positive test. A urine pregnancy test may produce a positive result as soon as 8 days after ovulation.

39. A B C D E

This is a favourite DRCOG topic.

According to the *British National Formulary* (BNF), the treatment for uncomplicated chlamydial infection is doxycycline 100 mg bd for 7 days. Erythromycin is used as an alternative drug during pregnancy. Chlamydial antigen and DNA may be detectable up to 3 weeks post-treatment. Chlamydial PID should be treated with an extended 14-day course of doxycycline.

40. A B C D E

This is a favourite DRCOG topic.

All are true. The perinatal mortality rate in the UK is ~9 per 1000 live and stillbirths.

41. A B C D E

This is a favourite DRCOG topic.

All are true. Causes of pruritus vulvae may be divided into general (systemic) and local. Systemic causes include Crohn's disease, skin diseases (psoriasis, lichen planus), polycythaemia, chronic liver and renal disease. Local causes include infestations, infections and vulval dystrophies (lichen sclerosus, leukoplakia and carcinoma).

42. A B C D E

This is a favourite DRCOG topic.

All are true. Causes of dyspareunia are divided into superficial and deep. Causes of superficial dyspareunia include atrophic vaginitis associated with the climacteric or oestrogen deficiency, lack of stimulation, postpartum perineal repair (suture, scar), ulceration, vaginismus, etc. Causes of deep dyspareunia include causes of chronic pelvic pain (endometriosis, infective pelvic inflammatory disease and pelvic congestion), and a fixed, retroverted uterus.

43. A B C E

This is a favourite DRCOG topic.

A serum β-hCG > 6000 IU l^{-1} is suggestive of an intrauterine pregnancy.

44. A B D E

This is a favourite DRCOG topic.

Procidentia is defined as a third-degree uterine prolapse or a complete prolapse of the uterus outside the vagina. Symptoms may include a dragging sensation with a lump lying outside the vulva, intermittent urinary retention, stress incontinence and difficulty in defecation. The exposed cervix may become ulcerated, infected and bleed. Most affected women are > 60 years of age. The condition is not commonly painful and is caused from laxity of the cardinal and uterosacral ligaments. The main predisposing factor is childbirth.

45. A B C

Management of procidentia is divided into conservative and surgical options. For the frail and elderly, topical oestrogen creams or a ring pessary are advised. Otherwise, a vaginal hysterectomy or a Fothergill (Manchester) repair is advocated. The latter preserves the uterus. A Fothergill repair involves amputation of the cervix, approximating the cardinal ligaments in front of the cervical stump to antevert the uterus, anterior colporrhaphy and posterior colpoperineorrhaphies.

46. A B C D E

All are true. Transplacental spread of CMV is associated with stillbirths, hepatosplenomegaly, microcephaly, chorioretinitis and thrombocytopaenia. *Toxoplasmosis gondii* acquired from uncooked meat or infected cat faeces may be transmitted transplacentally and result in cerebral calcification, chorioretinitis, epilepsy, microcephaly or hydrocephaly. Maternal rubella is also associated with congenital fetal anomalies.

47. A C D E

This is a favourite DRCOG topic.

Fetal and not maternal infection with rubella is diagnosed by chorionic villus sampling (CVS) from 8 to 11 weeks gestation. Cordocentesis on a fetal blood sample may also be performed at 18–20 weeks gestation to determine the presence of rubella-specific IgM antibodies. Contraction of maternal rubella during the first trimester is associated with a 70% incidence of congenital fetal abnormalities. The clinical manifestations of maternal rubella appear after a 14–21 day incubation and include posterior auricular, posterior cervical and suboccipital lymphadenopathy, mild fever and malaise, followed by a macular rash. Congenital fetal anomalies include cataracts, patent ductus arteriosus, sensorineural deafness, small for gestational age (SGA) neonate, microcephaly, mental retardation, thrombocytopaenic purpura, hepatosplenomegaly, jaundice, pneumonitis, pulmonic stenosis and ventricular septal defects.

48. A B D E

This is a favourite DRCOG topic.

Stage I is defined as disease limited to one or both ovaries. Stage II is defined as growth extending beyond the ovaries but confined to the pelvis. Stage III is classified as growth involving one or both ovaries with widespread intraperitoneal metastases. Stage IV is defined as disease with distant metastases. Ovarian carcinoma spreads locally and by lymphatic spread. It rarely spreads by the haematogenous route. As early ovarian cancer is symptomless, presentation usually occurs in Stage III and, therefore, results in a higher mortality rate than in cervical cancer. Management is surgical with a 6-month course of chemotherapy. However, the 5-year survival rate is still only 25%.

49. A C E

DUB is a diagnosis of exclusion and, therefore, cannot be caused by any organic pathology such as endometrial carcinoma. It occurs commonly in adolescence. Treatment may include medical (combined oral contraceptive (coc) pill, cyclical progestogens, NSAIDs, antifibrinolytic drugs, danazol, Mirena coil) or surgical (endometrial ablation or resection or hysterectomy) intervention.

50. A C D

Cow's milk contains more protein and calcium than breast milk. The calorific value of both is the same, however. Breast milk contains IgA, IgG, lactoferrin, lymphocytes and macrophages, which are protective against gastroenteritis. Cow's milk allergy presents with diarrhoea. Soya milk should then be substituted.

51. A E

Post-natal mastitis is caused by *Staphylococcus aureus* in 95% of cases. This is treated with flucloxacillin 250 mg o qds for 1 week. Breast-feeding is continued during antibiotic therapy. Infection occurs through a cracked nipple or blocked duct.

52. A B C D E

This is a favourite DRCOG topic.

All are true. Factors predisposing to PPH include retained placenta, a past history of uterine atony, high parity, prolonged labour, uterine anomaly or fibroids, polyhydramnios, twins, placental abruptio, pre-eclampsia, Caesarean section, placenta praevia, and clotting disorders (factor deficiencies or anticoagulant therapy).

53. A B D E

This is a favourite DRCOG topic.

ABO incompatibility is more common in mothers of blood group O. In these individuals, IgG and IgM antibodies may occur naturally, and the IgG antibodies may cross the placenta. Neonatal jaundice occurs within the first 24 hours of life, resulting in unconjugated hyperbilirubinaemia. A full blood count, mother and baby's blood group, and direct Coomb's test should be performed.

54. A B C D E

This is a favourite DRCOG topic.

All are true. Vaginal examination is contraindicated in the presence of suspected placenta praevia. A rhesus-negative mother should receive anti-D immunoglobulin with APH.

55. A D E

Turner's syndrome is 45XO. Edward's syndrome is trisomy 18.

56. B C D E

Primary amenorrhoea is defined as no menstruation by 14 years of age with absence of secondary sexual characteristics or no menstruation by 16 years of age with normal growth and sexual development. Any cause of secondary amenorrhoea can cause primary amenorrhoea.

57. A B D E

Chorio-amnionitis is caused by multiple organisms ascending from the cervix and vagina. Prolonged rupture of membranes is a risk factor. The clinical presentation is one of high maternal fever, fetal tachycardia and uterine irritability. A high vaginal swab should be taken and the mother should be started on systemic broad-spectrum antibiotics such as cefradine and metronidazole. Labour should be induced.

58. A C D E

Hydatidiform mole is associated with elevated β-hCG. Raised maternal serum α-fetoprotein may also be found with threatened abortion, teratoma, open neural tube defects and anencephaly.

59. A B C D E

All are true. Potter's syndrome comprises of fetal low-set ears, renal agenesis and hypoplastic lungs. Other causes of oligo-hydramnios include prolonged membrane rupture and placental insufficiency.

60. A B C D E

All are true. Intrauterine growth retardation (IUGR) is divided into symmetrical (due to chromosomal or intrauterine infection) or asymmetrical (due to placental insufficiency) types.

DRCOG OSCE for Circuit A
Questions

Station I
Interactive station

Instructions to candidates:

Mrs Collins is 28 years old and has been attempting to conceive for 3 years without success. Her GP has referred her to the out-patient gynaecology clinic. She now presents to you for advice. Take a gynaecological history.

This station lasts 6 minutes.

Station 2
Emergency contraception

1. Name the two types of emergency contraception pill? (2 marks)

2. What is the content and dose of each form of emergency contraceptive pill? (4 marks)

3. What is the effectiveness for each pill after 24 hours after unprotected intercourse? (2 marks)

4. What other form of emergency contraception can be offered? (1 mark)

5. Up to how many hours after unprotected sexual intercourse can this form of emergency contraception be offered? (1 mark)

Station 3
Interactive station

Instructions to candidates:

Miss Howe is a 22-year-old woman with two children and would like to be sterilized. She has a history of autoimmune hepatitis and has had a liver transplant. Obtain informed consent for tubal sterilization.

This station lasts 6 minutes.

Station 4
Down's syndrome

1. Name two types of screening tests for Down's syndrome? (2 marks)

2. At what gestation can these two screening tests be performed? (2 marks)

3. Name two types of diagnostic tests for Down's syndrome? (2 marks)

4. At what gestation can these two diagnostic tests be performed? (2 marks)

5. What is the risk of miscarriage for these two diagnostic tests? (2 marks)

Station 5
Interactive station

Instructions to candidates:

Mrs Sanderson is a 32-year-old woman who presents to the gynaecology clinic for advice after her third early miscarriage.

This station lasts 6 minutes.

Station 6

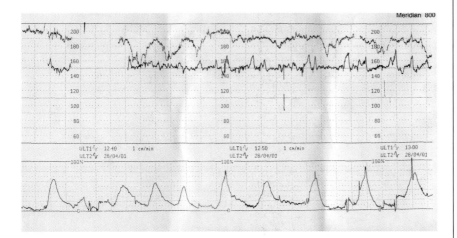

S. H. is a 27-year-old primigravid at 37 weeks' gestation.

1. What type of graph is depicted? (2 marks)

2. What is represented by each of the three tracings? (6 marks)

3. Is this graph normal, suspicious or ominous, and why? (1 mark)

4. What is the most appropriate form of management for the patient? (1 mark)

ANOMALY SCAN REPORT

Date: 1/03/2001   Visit 6

Patient:

Date of birth   5/11/1972

Menstrual cycle   Regular - LMP sure

Last menstrual period   : 31/07/2000

Gestation from LMP   : 30 wks + 3 days

Estimated date of delivery from LMP : 7/05/2001

Indication: Routine scan

Findings: **Twin pregnancy**

Fetus 1

Fetal measurements (plotted in relation to the normal mean ± 2 SDs)

Biparietal diameter	79.3 mm	├──•─┤
Head circumference	284.8 mm	├──•──┤
Abdominal circumference	254.2 mm	├─•─┤
Femur length	56.5 mm	├──•─┤
Head/Abdomen	1.120	├───•─┤

Gestational age by ultrasound   **30 + 3** weeks (EDD 5/05/2001)

Estimated fetal weight (US)   **1484 g**   ├──•──┤

Placenta   High anterior

Fetal presentation   Breech

Amniotic fluid volume   Normal

Fetus 2

Fetal measurements (plotted in relation to the normal mean ± 2 SDs)

Biparietal diameter	86.9 mm	├────•─┤
Head circumference	299.9 mm	├────•──┤
Abdominal circumference	255.4 mm	├──•───┤
Femur length	57.3 mm	├──•──┤
Head/Abdomen	1.174	├─────•─┤

Gestational age by ultrasound   **30 + 5** weeks (EDD 5/05/2001)

Estimated fetal weight (US)   **1592 g**   ├──•──┤

Placenta   High posterior

Fetal presentation   Breech

Amniotic fluid volume   Normal

1. What is of potential concern on the anomaly scan report? (1 mark)

2. If the condition persists, is vaginal delivery still feasible? (1 mark)

3. Under which condition may vaginal delivery be attempted? (1 mark)

4. Name four potential complications for which twins are more at risk than a singleton pregnancy? (4 marks)

5. Name three potential maternal complications in twin pregnancy? (3 marks)

Station 8
Urinary incontinence

Mrs Jones is a 50-year-old woman who presents with worsening urinary incontinence for the past 2 years. She states that it is worse when she coughs, sneezes or laughs. She denies frequency, urgency or nocturia. She has had three SVDs. Each child weighed 4.5, 4.0 and 3.7 kg respectively. She is now menopausal. She is not taking any medications. On examination, no prolapse is noted.

1. Name three investigations you can perform in a GP setting. (3 marks)

2. Name three investigations that can be arranged as an out-patient in hospital. (3 marks)

3. You have confirmed your suspicions. Name three medical treatment options you can offer the patient. (3 marks)

4. Name a surgical option for the patient if medical treatment fails. (1 mark)

Station 9

You are summoned by the midwife to see Mrs Yu who has just had a spontaneous vaginal delivery. Upon arrival, you see that she is lying in a pool of blood. You estimate she has lost 1–2 litres of blood.

1. What is the diagnosis? (1 mark)

2. Name four urgent actions you would take. (4 marks)

3. Name two drugs you would use for the patient. She is not hypertensive. (2 marks)

4. If she is hypertensive, what is the alternative drug treatment? (1 mark)

5. If the bleeding persists, which additional drug would you try? (1 mark)

6. Bleeding is not being controlled. What is the next line of management for the patient? (1 mark)

Station 10

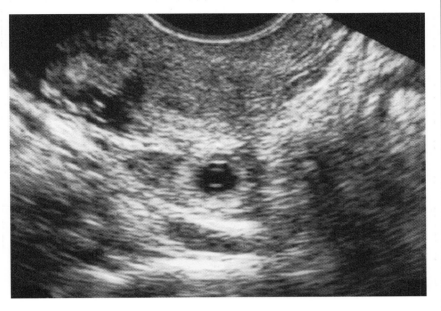

1. What is demonstrated on this transvaginal ultrasound picture? (1 mark)

2. What is the incidence of the condition? (1 mark)

3. Name three classic symptoms of the condition. (3 marks)

4. Name two predisposing factors for the condition. (2 marks)

5. How would you manage the patient? (3 marks)

Station 11

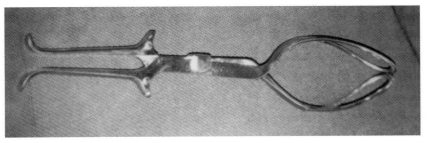

1. What is the name of the instrument? (1 mark)

2. In which circumstances is it used? (1 mark)

3. Name eight requirements that must be met for forceps delivery. (8 marks)

Station 12

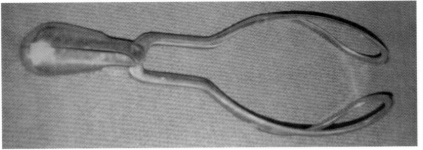

1. Name the instrument above. (1 mark)

2. In which circumstances is it used? (1 mark)

3. Name three reasons for this form of delivery. (3 marks)

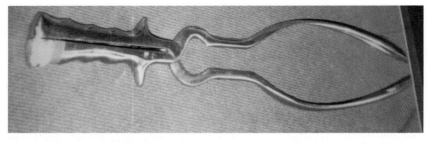

4. Name the instrument above. (1 mark)

5. In which circumstances would it be employed? (1 mark)

Station 13

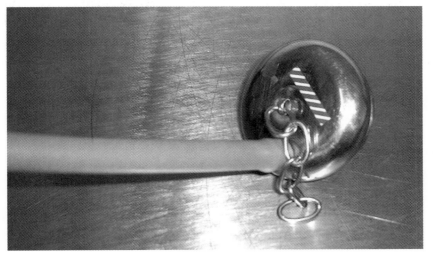

1. What is depicted above? (1 mark)

2. Name four advantages the instrument affords. (4 marks)

3. Name four potential complications associated with using the instrument. (4 marks)

Station 14

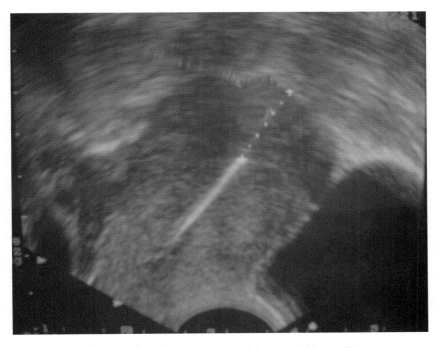

1. What is depicted in the ultrasound image? (1 mark)

2. What is its mechanism of action? (1 mark)

3. What are three contraindications to its use? (3 marks)

4. When in the cycle can it be inserted? (1 mark)

5. Name three possible complications that may be associated with its use. (3 marks)

6. For how many years is it effective? (1 mark)

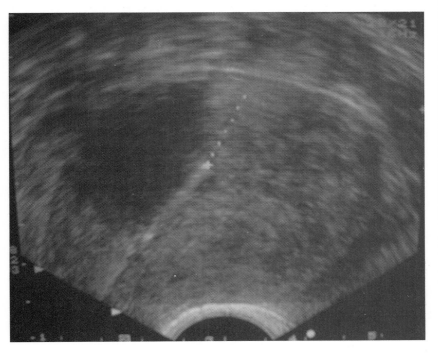

A 35-year-old woman is referred to you for lost threads of her Mirena coil. You are unable to see the threads on speculum examination and perform a transvaginal ultrasound.

1. What do you tell the patient from the ultrasound image? (1 mark)

2. What is the active component of a Mirena intrauterine system (IUS)? (1 mark)

3. Name three actions of the IUS. (3 marks)

4. Name two advantages the IUS has over the intrauterine contraceptive device. (2 marks)

5. Name two disadvantages the IUS has over the IUCD. (2 marks)

6. How many years is the IUS licensed for use in the UK before it has to be replaced? (1 mark)

Station 16

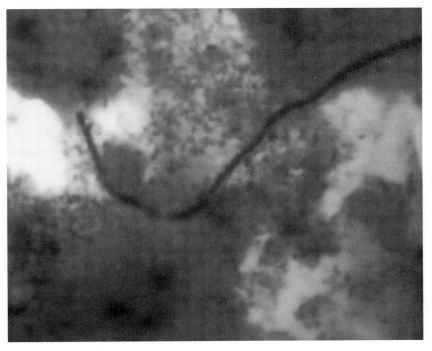

A 24-year-old woman presents with foul-smelling vaginal discharge. You perform a speculum examination and take swabs for microscopy, culture and sensitivities.

1. What abnormal morphology is shown on the slide? (2 marks)

2. What are the names of the two concurrent infections? (2 marks)

3. Are these infections always sexually transmitted? (1 mark)

4. Name three risk factors for acquiring either disease. (3 marks)

5. What is the treatment for each condition? (2 marks)

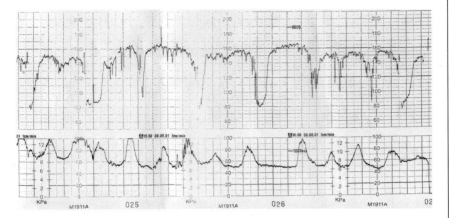

A. H. is a 26-year-old para 0 39/40 who is actively contracting. On examination, she is 6 cm dilated.

1. What type of graph is depicted? (2 marks)

2. What is the fetal baseline heart rate? Is this normal? (2 marks)

3. What is the fetal baseline variability? Is this normal? (2 marks)

4. Is this graph normal, suspicious or ominous, and why? (2 marks)

5. What is the most appropriate form of management for the patient? (2 marks)

Station 18

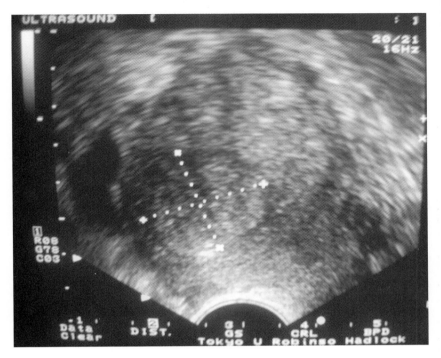

K. S. is a 40-year-old woman who presents with menorrhagia and dysmenorrhoea.

1. What is depicted in the transvaginal ultrasound? (1 mark)

2. Is there cause for alarm? (1 mark)

3. In what three positions can this mass be found? (3 marks)

4. Which type is most likely to be symptomatic? (1 mark)

5. What medical treatments can be offered to the patient? (2 marks)

6. What is the surgical treatment for the condition? What is offered as pre-operative treatment? (2 marks)

Station 19

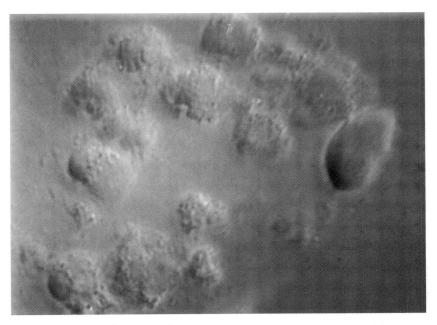

C. C. is a 22-year-old woman who complains of post-coital bleeding and frothy vaginal discharge.

1. What is the organism depicted on the slide? (1 mark)

2. On what type of mount has the specimen been placed? (1 mark)

3. At what pH does this organism thrive? (1 mark)

4. What would you expect to find on speculum examination of the cervix? (1 mark)

5. Is this a sexually transmitted disease? (1 mark)

6. What is the treatment for this disease? (1 mark)

7. What must you warn the patient when prescribing this drug? (1 mark)

8. What three things must you advise the patient to do before you send her away? (3 marks)

Station 20

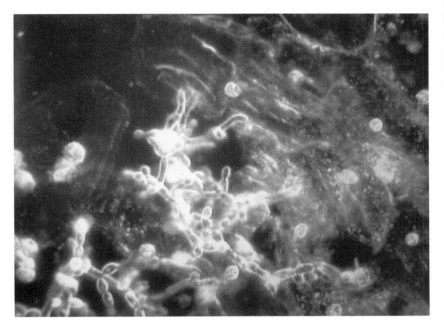

K. M. is a 26-year-old woman who presents to the GUM clinic complaining of a painless ulcer on her vulva.

1. What type of examination is depicted? (1 mark)

2. What organism is depicted? (1 mark)

3. Is this primary or secondary? (1 mark)

4. How was the specimen obtained? (1 mark)

5. Name three serologic tests for the disease. (3 marks)

6. What is the treatment for the disease? (1 mark)

7. What may occur within hours after treatment is commenced? (1 mark)

8. How is this reaction managed? (1 mark)

DRCOG OSCE for Circuit B
Questions

Station 1

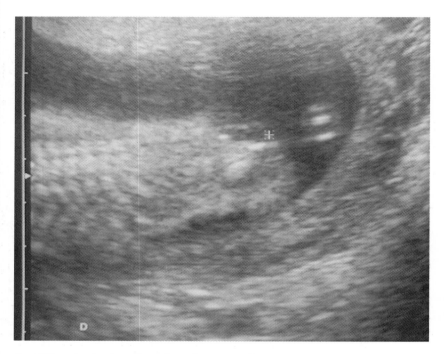

1. What is depicted in the ultrasound image? (1 mark)

2. What marker is used for open neural tube defects? (1 mark)

3. Name the four subdivisions of the condition. (4 marks)

4. Name four associated problems the infant may develop. (4 marks)

Station 2
Interactive station

Instructions to candidates:

Mrs Thomas is a 24-year-old woman who presents with PV spotting at 29/40. Discuss the management of the patient with the examiner.

This station lasts 6 minutes.

Station 3

Miss Cooper is a 22-year-old para 0 who is 18 weeks pregnant and complains of lower abdominal pain for the past 2 days. Her blood pressure is 110/80 and her pulse rate is 90 bpm.

1. What is your initial management for the patient? (1 mark)

2. What four things would you perform on clinical examination? (4 marks)

3. What three investigations would you arrange for the patient? (3 marks)

4. Her urine dipstick is positive for nitrates and leukocytes. Which antibiotic would you prescribe? (1 mark)

5. What is an alternative choice if she is penicillin-allergic? (1 mark)

Station 4

Miss Wood is a 14-year-old girl who complains of painful periods that interfere with school. Her mother adds that she has temper tantrums and is extremely irritable before her periods. She is present with her mother.

1. What is the diagnosis for her painful periods? (1 mark)

2. Name three possible premenstrual symptoms. (3 marks)

3. Name two medical treatments for premenstrual tension. (2 marks)

4. What two questions would you inquire of the daughter away from her mother? (2 marks)

5. Name two treatment options you would offer this young girl. (2 marks)

Station 5

Mrs Akintillo has just delivered a 28-week stillborn by normal vaginal delivery.

1. Name three of the seven blood investigations you would obtain of the mother. (3 marks)

2. What other maternal investigation would you obtain? (1 mark)

3. What instructions would you give about the placenta? (1 mark)

4. Name the five options for post-mortem. (5 marks)

Station 6

Mrs K. Adams is a 35-year-old para 3 who is 21 weeks pregnant. She presents to you as she has wet the bed. She is concerned.

1. What is the most likely diagnosis? (1 mark)

2. What questions would you ask of the patient? (3 marks)

3. What three things would you perform on clinical examination? (3 marks)

4. What investigations would you perform? (2 marks)

5. You confirm your suspicions on speculum exam. What is the prognosis for this pregnancy? (1 mark)

Station 7

Miss L. Lane is a 34-year-old woman who presents to Casualty with sudden onset of severe, constant, right-sided iliac fossa pain. Her temperature is 39°C, her blood pressure 108/80 and her pulse rate is 90 bpm. She feels nauseous. Both her urine pregnancy and urine dipstick tests are negative. She had a coil fitted 2 months before. On abdominal examination, you are told she has peritoneal signs. However, the surgical team thinks it unlikely she has acute appendicitis. They ask you, the Gynaecology SHO, to give an opinion.

1. Name three likely findings on bimanual, PV and speculum examination. (3 marks)

2. On speculum examination, the threads of the coil are clearly visible. Would you remove the coil? (1 mark)

3. What is the most likely diagnosis? (1 mark)

4. Name three investigations you would perform to confirm the diagnosis. (3 marks)

5. What treatment would you offer the patient? (1 mark)

6. How would you alter the above treatment in a pregnant patient? (1 mark)

Station 8
Interactive station

Instructions to candidates:

Miss A. Jefferson is a 24-year-old woman who presents with a 6-month history of irregular menstrual cycles and heavy periods. Take a gynaecological history. What initial treatment would you offer Miss Jefferson?

This station lasts 6 minutes.

Station 9
Interactive station

Instructions to candidates:

Miss A. Lyons has received a contact card to attend the GUM clinic. She decided to see you, the GP, instead. She tells you she is 8 weeks pregnant. Explain to the examiner the advice you would offer the patient as to why she should still attend the GUM clinic.

This station lasts 6 minutes.

Station 10
Interactive station

Instructions to candidates:

Mrs K. Everett is a 31-year-old woman who would like to have her first baby. She presents to you for advice. Offer the patient some pre-conception advice.

This station lasts 6 minutes.

Station 11

Miss L. Marks is a 36-year-old woman who presents to Casualty with sudden onset of severe, left-sided, iliac fossa pain and PV spotting. She explains that she was sterilized 1 year ago. She is rhesus-negative. Her temperature is 37°C, her blood pressure is 100/60 and her pulse rate is 98 bpm. Her urine hCG is positive. The Casualty Officer has inserted a venflon and taken blood for full blood count and group and save.

1. Name three possible diagnoses. (3 marks)

2. On PV examination, the cervical os is long and closed with prune juice-coloured PV spotting. There is left-sided adnexal tenderness. What investigation would you arrange urgently? (½ mark)

3. The above investigation fails to locate a pregnancy. Which two blood tests would you arrange? (2 marks)

4. The blood test results come back as hCG = 1200 IU l⁻¹ and progesterone = 65 nmol l⁻¹. What does this suggest about her pregnancy? (½ mark)

5. What action would you take for the patient in light of the above findings? (½ mark)

6. Name three treatment options for this condition. (3 marks)

7. Does the patient need anti-D immunoglobulin? (½ mark)

Station 12

Miss P. Parker is a 20-year-old woman who presents to the GUM clinic with a contact card. She states she has copious yellow-green vaginal discharge and is 6 weeks pregnant.

1. What is the most likely diagnosis? (1 mark)

2. Name two complications of this disease. (2 marks)

3. What is another possible diagnosis? (1 mark)

4. Name four locations where swabs can be taken to exclude this sexually transmitted disease. (4 marks)

5. Can this organism be identified on a Gram-stain? (1 mark)

6. What treatment would you offer the patient? (1 mark)

Station 13
Interactive station

Instructions to candidates:

You receive a cervical smear report for Mrs Stanton that shows severe dyskaryosis. Explain to the patient her results and the coloposcopy procedure.

This station lasts 6 minutes.

Station 14

Mrs S. Saunders is a 37-year-old woman who presents with inter-menstrual bleeding. She smokes a packet of cigarettes a day and weighs 100 kg. She is 1.60 m tall. Her periods are regular (28-day cycle) but last for 7–10 days. She describes her periods as so heavy that she cannot leave the house for fear of drenching her clothes. She currently uses the natural method for contraception and has four children. She has come to you for help about her IMB and menorrhagia and for a better form of contraception.

1. Name four investigations you can do in the Outpatient Clinic? (4 marks)

2. For which investigation would you refer her and when in her cycle? (1 mark)

3. Which form of contraception is contraindicated in her situation? (1 mark)

4. Name two options for contraception that will also manage her IMB and menorrhagia. (2 marks)

5. What are her surgical options? (2 marks)

Station 15

Mrs P. Smith is a 44-year-old woman who presents with irregular menstrual cycles, weight gain, hair loss and brittle nails. Her LMP was 3 months ago. Her initial blood investigation is as follows:

LH: 35 IU l^{-1}

FSH: 45 IU l^{-1}

Oestradiol: 65 pmol l^{-1}

1. What is the diagnosis? (1 mark)

2. Name five symptoms. (5 marks)

3. Name three forms of treatment. (3 marks)

4. How would treatment alter if the patient had had a hysterectomy? (1 mark)

Station 16

Mrs J. Osborne is a 35-year-old woman who has just delivered a term baby boy and wishes to breast-feed.

1. Name three advantages breast-feeding offers the baby. (3 marks)

2. Name three advantages breast-feeding offers the mother. (3 marks)

3. Name three conditions for the lactational amenorrhoea method of contraception. (3 marks)

4. What is her chance of pregnancy with the lactational amenorrhoea method if all the conditions are met? (1 mark)

Station 17

Mrs E. Marsland is a 24-year-old para 1 who presents at 28/40 with premature contractions.

1. Name five causes of preterm labour. (5 marks)

2. How would you assess the patient? (3 marks)

3. Which agents would you administer and why? (2 marks)

Station 18

Mrs F. Patel is a 38-year-old woman who has been referred to the gynaecology clinic for chronic right-sided pelvic pain. She has never had any surgical operations. She states that the pain is worse after she has opened her bowels, after exercise and after intercourse. The pain is better with application of heat to her abdomen. On examination, pain is elicited one-third the distance from the iliac crest to the umbilicus.

1. Name three gynaecological causes of chronic pelvic pain, placing the most likely diagnosis first. (3 marks)

2. What investigation would you perform in the Outpatient Clinic? (1 mark)

3. Name three investigations you would arrange for the patient. (3 marks)

4. Name three forms of treatment for the patient. (3 marks)

Station 19

Miss A. Lange is a 28-year-old obese woman who is having difficulty conceiving. She also complains of pelvic pain, dysmenorrhoea, dyspareunia and dyschesia. Her cycles come every 21 days and last for 10 days.

1. What is the most likely diagnosis? (1 mark)

2. Name three investigations for the condition. (3 marks)

3. Name three forms of medical treatment for the condition. (3 marks)

4. Name three forms of surgical treatment for the condition. (3 marks)

Station 20

Mr and Mrs Wilson are keen to have a baby but have been unable to conceive for 3 years. Mr Wilson provides a seminal fluid sample. His SFA is as follows:

Volume: 1.5 ml

Density: 10×10^6 ml^{-1}

Motility: 35% progressively motile

Morphology: 25% normal

1. What is the name for each of the patient's seminal fluid analysis abnormalities? (4 marks)

2. Name three other investigations for male infertility. (3 marks)

3. Name three options for the couple, assuming Mrs Wilson is fertile. (3 marks)

DRCOG OSCE for Circuit C
Questions

Station 1

Mrs Brown is a 28-year-old para 1 who is 36 weeks pregnant. She calls the labour ward and informs you that she has dark green vaginal discharge. She is not contracting.

1. What do you suspect has occurred, and what do you advise her to do next? (2 marks)

2. On examination, you confirm your suspicions. The CTG shows a baseline fetal heart rate of 140 bpm with good variability. There are no uterine contractions. How would you next manage the patient? (1 mark)

3. On VE, her cervical os allows a fingertip. What medication would you administer to the patient? (1 mark)

4. Name two potential implications of significant fresh meconium in the amniotic fluid. (2 marks)

5. Six hours later, her cervix is 6 cm dilated, with vigorous uterine contractions. The CTG now shows persistent variable decelerations with shouldering and a baseline rate of 170 bpm. Name two options for management. (2 marks)

6. Name four possible complications associated with a Caesarean section. (2 marks)

Station 2

Mrs Bradshaw delivered a baby boy by traumatic forceps delivery 2 weeks before. She complains of tearfulness, depression, worthlessness, inability to breast-feed and difficulty sleeping.

1. What do you suspect she has? (1 mark)

2. Name three aetiological factors. (3 marks)

3. Name three symptoms that would make you suspect puerperal psychosis. (3 marks)

4. If you suspected a diagnosis of puerperal psychosis, which two classes of drugs are recommended for the treatment of her condition? (2 marks)

5. Which location would you select to treat the mother? (1 mark)

Station 3

Mrs Morgan is a 58-year-old woman who presents to Casualty with acute onset of profuse PV bleed with passage of clots. She states she reached menopause 10 years before.

1. Name three possible causes for her PVB. (3 marks)

2. How would you manage the patient in Casualty? (5 marks)

3. What two investigations would you arrange for the patient? (2 marks)

Station 4

Mrs Collins has IDDM and presents for her first Antenatal Clinic appointment.

1. Which test is used to confirm diabetes? (1 mark)

2. What will happen to the patient's insulin requirements during her pregnancy? (1 mark)

3. Name three maternal complications of diabetic pregnancy. (3 marks)

4. Name four fetal complications of diabetic pregnancy. (4 marks)

5. How would you plan to deliver the patient's baby? (1 mark)

Station 5

Miss James is a 27-year-old woman who complains of amenorrhoea for 6 months and weight gain. Her urine β-hCG is negative. You arrange for serum hormonal levels and are presented with the following results:

Oestradiol: 350 pmol l⁻¹

FSH: 5 IU l⁻¹

LH: 15 IU l⁻¹

Testosterone: 5 nmol l⁻¹

1. What is the most likely diagnosis? (1 mark)

2. Name four symptoms or signs associated with this condition. (4 marks)

3. What investigation would you arrange to confirm the diagnosis? (1 mark)

4. What medical treatment would you offer the patient if she plans to conceive? (1 mark)

5. How would your management alter if the patient does not plan to conceive in the near future? (1 mark)

6. Name two surgical treatments for the condition. (2 marks)

Station 6
Interactive station

Instructions to candidates:

Miss Whittam is a 19-year-old woman who has just had a TOP. She comes to you to discuss contraception. Offer the patient advice about her hormonal contraceptive options.

This station lasts 6 minutes.

Station 7

Mrs Lim is a 19-year-old primip who is 28 weeks pregnant. Her blood pressure is taken in the Antenatal Clinic and is 170/110. On urine dipstick, she has 2+ proteins. She complains of frontal headache and nausea.

1. What is the diagnosis? (1 mark)

2. Name three associated symptoms and signs. (3 marks)

3. How would you manage the patient? (1 mark)

4. Name four investigations you would arrange urgently. (4 marks)

5. Which drug would you administer to control the patient's blood pressure? (1 mark)

Station 8
Pearl Index

1. What is the definition of the Pearl Index? (1 mark)

2. How is it calculated? (1 mark)

3. What is the Pearl Index for male or female sterilization? (1 mark)

4. What is the Pearl Index for the progestogen-only pill? (1 mark)

5. What is the Pearl Index for the combined oral contraceptive? (1 mark)

6. What is the Pearl Index for the Depo-Provera injection? (1 mark)

7. What is the Pearl Index for the Mirena intrauterine system? (1 mark)

8. What is the Pearl Index for the Multiload Cu 375 intrauterine device? (1 mark)

9. What is the Pearl Index for the lactational amenorrhoea method? (1 mark)

10. What is the Pearl Index for the cervical cap with spermicide? (1 mark)

Station 9
Interactive station

Instructions to candidates:

Mrs White is a 40-year-old woman who is concerned that she may be at risk for having a Down's syndrome baby. She is 8 weeks pregnant. Discuss her risk and describe the two screening tests and the two diagnostic tests for Down's syndrome. Allay her fears.

This station lasts 6 minutes.

Station 10
Interactive station

Instructions to candidates:

Mrs Wilson is a 50-year-old woman who has come to you to discuss hormone-replacement therapy (HRT). Explain to the examiner the pros and cons of HRT, the different forms of HRT and the cost implications to the NHS.

This station lasts 6 minutes.

Station 11

You are presented with a 3-week-old baby who is still jaundiced.

1. Name five tests you would arrange urgently. (5 marks)

2. Name five causes for this prolonged neonatal jaundice. (5 marks)

Mrs Hanks is a 30-year-old woman who is separated with four children. Her BMI is 40. She has been in a new relationship for the past 3 months and comes to you requesting a reversal of her laparoscopic sterilization.

1. Name three reasons why she is not a suitable candidate. (3 marks)

2. Name four suggestions you would make. (4 marks)

3. What is the success rate for reversal of laparoscopic sterilization? (1 mark)

4. What can you inform the patient about the cost of such a procedure and what is her alternative option? (2 marks)

Station 13

You are asked to attend a home birth. Your concern is that the mother is high risk and refuses to attend the hospital.

1. What are the five signs that are assessed in Apgar scoring? (5 marks)

2. At what times are they taken? (1 mark)

3. The baby has apnoea, persistent cyanosis and a heart rate of 90 bpm. Name two actions you would take. (2 marks)

4. At how many breaths per minute would you ventilate the baby? (1 mark)

5. The baby's heart rate is dropping to 55 bpm. At what compression:ventilation ratio would you administer chest compressions? (1 mark)

Station 14

Mrs Johnson is a 20-year-old primigravida who presents in labour. On vaginal examination, she is 6 cm dilated and contracting regularly. Four hours later, she is still 6 cm dilated. Her uterine contractions are now irregular.

1. What has happened? (1 mark)

2. Name three reasons for this to have occurred. (3 marks)

3. What is your next action? (1 mark)

4. It has now been 8 hours and the cervix is still only 6 cm dilated. What is your next course of action? (1 mark)

5. How would your management differ in a multigravida? (1 mark)

6. If on arrival, the patient's cervix had been effaced but not dilated, how long would you wait to intervene? (1 mark)

7. What is this condition called and how would you intervene? (2 marks)

Station 15
Female urinary incontinence

1. Name three causes of genuine stress incontinence. (3 marks)

2. Name three forms of treatment for stress incontinence. (3 marks)

3. Name two causes of detrusor instability. (2 marks)

4. Name two forms of treatment for detrusor instability. (2 marks)

BIPARIETAL DIAMETER (Outer-inner)
3rd, 10th, 50th, 90th and 97th centiles

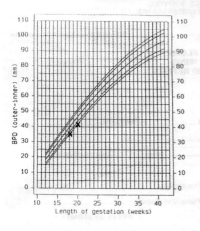

HEAD CIRCUMFERENCE (plotted)
3rd, 10th, 50th, 90th and 97th centiles

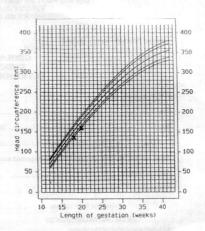

FEMUR
3rd, 10th, 50th, 90th and 97th centiles

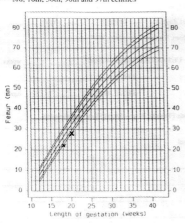

ABDOMINAL CIRCUMFERENCE (plotted)
3rd, 10th, 50th, 90th and 97th centiles

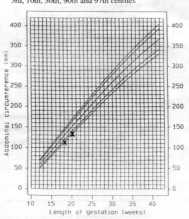

1. What is shown on the ultrasound scan report? Assume the fetus has a normal amniotic fluid volume. (1 mark)

2. Name five causes for the condition. (5 marks)

3. Name two investigations you would arrange. (2 marks)

4. Name two forms of fetal monitoring other than serial ultra-sounds. (2 marks)

Station 17
Cervical screening

1. At which age group is cervical screening targeted? (1 mark)

2. When in the cycle should the smear test be taken? (1 mark)

3. Name three risk factors for cervical cancer. (3 marks)

4. Name three indications for referral for colposcopy. (3 marks)

5. Name two methods of treatment of cervical intraepithelial neoplasia (CIN). (2 marks)

Mrs Grant is a 30-year-old mother of three who comes to you for advice about contraception. She suffers from epilepsy for which she takes carbamazepine. She does not smoke. Her BMI = 25. She also adds that she has had breakthrough bleeding with her current combined oral contraceptive pill (coc) logynon. Her smear was taken 6 months ago and was normal.

1. Name three possible causes for her breakthrough bleeding. (3 marks)

2. Name three other enzyme-inducers. (3 marks)

3. Name three options for contraception for the patient. (3 marks)

4. If she were to conceive in the future, what advice would you need to offer the patient about carbamazepine? (1 mark)

Station 19

Miss Stanton is a 15-year-old girl who presents to you for emergency contraception. She states that she had missed pill numbers 3 and 4 in her Marvelon packet and has had sexual intercourse the night before.

1. Is she a candidate for emergency contraception? (1 mark)

2. If she had missed two pills from the last seven in her packet, would she be a candidate for emergency contraception? (1 mark)

3. Can she legally give consent for medical treatment? (1 mark)

4. What would you offer and advise the patient? (3 marks)

5. She returns and states that she had unprotected sexual intercourse 1 week ago. You calculate that sexual intercourse took place on day 13 of her cycle. You look at her Marvelon packet and note she has missed four pills mid-packet (days 12–15). What would you offer and advise her now? (3 marks)

6. What is the mechanism of action of the IUD? (1 mark)

Station 20
Postpartum contraception

Mrs Smith is a 20-year-old woman who has delivered a baby boy 6 weeks before and would like to be started on the combined oral contraceptive (coc) pill.

1. What key piece of information do you need to know? (1 mark)

2. If she was not breast-feeding, when should she have started the coc? (1 mark)

3. If she is breast-feeding, what are her choices for contraception? (4 marks)

4. She chooses the POP. When in her cycle would you start her on the POP and what advice would you offer her? (3 marks)

Miss Marks is a 19-year-old woman who has undergone a TOP and is ready for discharge. She states that she has difficulty remembering to take the pill.

5. What form of contraception would you offer and administer before discharge? (1 mark)

DRCOG OSCE for Circuit A
Answers

Station 1: Answers

The examiner and the patient (a role-playing actress) will be marking you out of ten possible points, with one point assigned to each of the following points:

1. **Establishing rapport:** introduce yourself to the patient in a friendly manner. Smile, greet her by name and shake her hand. 'Welcome to the gynaecology clinic Mrs Collins.'

2. **Verbal/non-verbal cues:** do you pick up cues given by the patient?

3. **Eye contact:** do you maintain good eye contact with the patient?

4. **Take a gynaecological history:** ideally, both partners should be present. Specific gynaecological questions include: When was her menarche? When was her last menstrual period? Are her periods regular? Does she have a 28- or 35-day cycle? How many days do her periods last? Are they heavy? Does she pass clots? Has she ever been pregnant? Does she have a history of ectopics or miscarriages? Does she have a history of any gynaecological operations or illnesses? When was her last cervical smear? Has it ever been abnormal?

5. **Other relevant history:** other pertinent questions include the couple's ages, occupations, i.e. any history of exposure to environmental hazards or chemical toxins, social habits, such as frequency and amount of drinking or binge drinking, smoking habits, frequency of sexual intercourse, and any history of sexually transmitted diseases.

6. **Avoidance of medical jargon.**

7. **Inform the patient of her options in layman's terms:** explain to her that both she and her partner should undergo testing. Her husband would need to supply a semen analysis after 3–5 days of abstinence. The specimen should be brought to the laboratory immediately for analysis. He may need to repeat the semen analysis if the sample is not cleared. Her blood tests include FSH and LH, preferably on day 5 of her cycle, oestrogen, sex hormone-binding globulin, prolactin and progesterone level on day 21 of her cycle if she has a 28-day cycle. She should also be offered a transvaginal pelvic ultrasound.

8. **Allow the patient to ask questions:** ask the patient if you have explained things clearly or would she like you to clarify?

9. **Give the patient a follow-up appointment:** in this case, advise the patient to make an appointment at the front desk for 6 weeks' time to return for the results.

10. **Would the patient like to see you again?**

The role-playing actress has the option to give you an extra point.

Station 2: Answers

This is a favourite DRCOG OSCE topic.

1. The two types of emergency contraceptive pill recommended by the RCOG and the Faculty of Family Planning and Reproductive Health Care are Levonelle-2 and Schering PC4.

2. The content and dose of Levonelle-2 is two tablets, each containing a 750-mcg dose of levonorgestrel. The first dose must be taken within 72 hours of unprotected intercourse, the second tablet being taken 12 hours later. The content and dose of Schering PC4 consists of four tablets, each containing 50 mcg ethinyloestradiol and 500 mcg norgestrel. Two tablets are taken within 72 hours of unprotected intercourse and the remaining two tablets are taken 12 hours later.

3. Levonelle-2 is 95% effective if taken within 24 hours of unprotected intercourse. Schering PC-4 is 77% effective if taken within 24 hours of unprotected intercourse. The emergency contraceptive pill is effective within 72 hours of unprotected intercourse but efficacy falls to 58% for Levonelle-2 and 31% for Schering PC-4.

4. The intrauterine emergency contraception is an alternative method.

5. The IUD can be offered within 5 days of unprotected intercourse or up to 5 days after the calculated earliest day of ovulation, i.e. day 19 of a 28-day shortest cycle. The patient should be warned of side-effects such as heavy or more painful periods, perforation of the uterus, displacement and risk of post-insertion pelvic infection. If the patient has more than one partner per year, she should be screened for STDs and offered doxycycline at 100 mg bd for 1 week.

This is a favourite DRCOG OSCE topic.

Guidelines to counselling can be obtained from http://www.jhuccp.org/pr/j48/counsel.stm. These guidelines suggest using the mnemonic 'GATHER'.

1. **Greet** the patient and introduce yourself.

2. **Ask** the patient what her reasons are for opting for tubal sterilization. Ask her about her partner and whether he has considered a vasectomy, which is a safer option and can be performed under a local anaesthetic.

3. **Tell** the patient about her alternative options. In the patient's case, as she has had a healthy liver transplant, her liver is no longer diseased and she can take the combined oral contraceptive (coc) pill without fear of increased first-pass hepatic metabolism in a diseased liver. Explain that other options include:

   - Implanon is a contraceptive implant that is inserted under the skin of the inner upper arm and lasts for 3 years. It is 99% effective.

   - Depo-Provera or Noristerat contraceptive injections last for 12 and 8 weeks, respectively, and are 99% effective.

   - IUD (in view of her liver transplant, this form of contraception, i.e. a foreign body in the uterus, may not be her first choice).

4. Tell the patient about the **risks and benefits** of tubal sterilization:

   - It is a surgical procedure with all the inherent risks of a general anaesthetic. There is a 1 in 10 000 risk of death from a general anaesthetic.

   - The procedure is usually performed laparoscopically (keyhole surgery) but may need to be converted to a mini-laparotomy and thus leave a bigger surgical scar.

   - The procedure has a 1 in 200 lifetime risk of failure.

   - Early complications include a < 5% risk of bleeding, infection or trauma to the organs and there is a small risk of late complication of ectopic pregnancy.

- It is permanent and consequently there is a risk of regret as she is only 22 years old and may not be ready for permanent sterilization, especially if she finds a new partner. She must understand that her family will now be complete. Ideally, suitable patients for this operation are > 35 years of age.

5. **Stress the cost–benefit aspect of this procedure.** Points in the DRCOG exam are awarded if this issue is brought up:

   - Reversal of the procedure costs £2500 and may not be available on the NHS. The success rate of the reversal operation ranges from 25 to 70% depending on the surgeon and whether a microscope is employed. Alternatively, IVF (*in-vitro* fertilization) treatments are expensive and, again, not available on the NHS.

   - The benefit is that the patient will be sterilized permanently. It is a single procedure and relatively safe. It is highly effective.

6. **Help** her decide. Ask if she has understood everything or needs clarification.

7. **Explain** the procedure. Through keyhole surgery, i.e. a cut below the umbilicus, her tubes will be permanently clipped with Filschie clips.

8. **Return** for follow-up. She may need time to digest all you have discussed. Offer her another appointment if she would like to discuss the consent form with her partner in detail before signing the form.

Station 4: Answers

This is a favourite DRCOG OSCE topic.

1. The two screening tests for Down's syndrome are the measurement of the nuchal fold thickness on ultrasound and the triple blood test for serum oestriol, α-fetoprotein and β-human chorionic gonadotrophin (hCG).

2. The nuchal fold thickness scan is performed at 11–14 weeks' gestation; the triple blood test can be performed at 14–16 weeks' gestation.

3. The two diagnostic tests for Down's syndrome are chorionic villus sampling (CVS) and amniocentesis.

4. CVS is performed at 10 weeks. Testing any sooner would carry a high risk of limb malformations in the fetus. Amniocentesis is performed at 16 weeks' gestation.

5. The risk of miscarriage for CVS is 1 in 20; the risk of miscarriage for amniocentesis is 1 in 200. This hot topic may also appear in the DRCOG exam as an interactive station, so be prepared to describe the procedures to a role-playing mother.

Station 5: Answers

This is a favourite DRCOG OSCE topic.

1. **Greet** the patient, introduce yourself and sympathize with her recent miscarriage.

2. **Inform** the patient that after three miscarriages it would be a good idea to investigate the reasons for her recurrent miscarriages (RM). This diagnosis can only be made after three documented miscarriages at < 24 weeks' gestation with no more than one living child from the current partnership.

3. **Ask her about her three miscarriages.** At what gestation: first or second trimester losses? Were they all with the same partner? How many living children are there? If the miscarriage occurred in the second trimester, the length of her cervix can be measured by ultrasound at 12–14 weeks' gestation when she is next pregnant and cervical cerclage offered if she has cervical incompetence. The Shirodkhar suture is then removed at 37 weeks' gestation.

4. **Take a complete gynaecological history.** Ask questions about her onset of menarche, length and regularity of her menses, her last cervical smear and the result. Ask her about any prior history of gynaecological operations especially to the cervix. Cone biopsy has been associated with RM. Ask about any prior history of STDs or PID. Ask her about her social habits of alcohol intake and smoking, and her occupation. Ask about any pre-existing illnesses or medical conditions. Diabetes mellitus and thyroid disease have both been associated with RM.

5. **Offer her options for blood testing for maternal antibodies.** She can be tested for lupus anticoagulant, antiphospholipid antibodies and anticardiolipin antibodies. Up to 30% of first trimester RM harbour antiphospholipid antibodies.

6. **Offer her blood testing and a transvaginal pelvic ultrasound for polycystic ovary syndrome.** The level of LH can be three times that of FSH in PCO. Up to 56% of women with RM have polycystic ovaries. Take blood at day 5 of the cycle for LH, FSH, and testosterone.

7. **Suggest** that both partners have **chromosomal analysis** to exclude balanced translocation.

8. **Check rubella status.**

9. **Offer the patient a haemoglobinopathy screen** if she or her partner are in a high-risk group.

10. **Offer the patient a hysterosalpingogram** to exclude cervical incompetence or uterine anomaly such as bicornuate uterus. Hysteroscopy may be booked as a daycase if the hysterosalpingogram or transvaginal ultrasound is suspect.

Station 6: Answers

1. It is a cardiotocograph.

2. The first two tracings are of twins 1 and 2. The lower tracing is recording the maternal contractions.

3. This CTG is ominous. It depicts prolonged fetal tachycardia in twin 1 with a baseline heart rate of 190 bpm and the presence of late decelerations, both indications of hypoxia. Normal baseline heart rate should be between 110 and 150 bpm.

4. Appropriate management for the patient would be to proceed to emergency Caesarean section.

Station 7: Answers

1. A potential concern is the breech presentation in both twins.

2. If this persists, the twins will need to be delivered by Caesarean section.

3. Only if the lower-lying twin has a cephalic presentation during labour can vaginal delivery be attempted. The position of the higher lying twin has no bearing on vaginal delivery.

4. Potential fetal complications of twin pregnancy include twin-to-twin transfusion, intrauterine growth retardation (IUGR), increased incidence of congenital anomalies, polyhydramnios, malpresentation, premature labour and increased abortion rate.

5. Potential maternal complications of twin pregnancy include anaemia, gestational diabetes, pre-eclampsia and postpartum haemorrhage.

Station 8: Answers

This is a favourite DRCOG OSCE topic.

1. The three investigations that can be performed at a GP setting include urine dipstick for glucose to exclude diabetes, midstream urine for microscopy and culture, and offering the patient a frequency volume chart to record hourly intake and output over 24 hours and during periods of incontinence. The pad test is now obsolete. This test entails weighing a pad pre- and post-daily wear.

2. The three investigations that can be arranged as an outpatient in hospital include a pelvic ultrasound to exclude fibroids, and basic urodynamic investigations such as uroflowmetry and cystometry. Uroflowmetry involves the patient urinating on a flow meter and measuring how quickly the bottom is filled. Normal flow rate is $15\,ml\ s^{-1}$ for $>150\,ml$. Cystometry measures rectal, bladder, and detrusor pressures and flow.

3. You have confirmed your suspicions of genuine stress incontinence. Risk factors include congenital weakness such as Ehlers–Danlos, pregnancy, vaginal delivery of heavy infants, menopause due to deficiency in oestrogen and previous incontinence surgery. The medical options for treatment include pelvic floor exercises, vaginal cones, electrical stimulation to increase the pelvic floor muscles, wearing a tampon to hold up the urethra during exercise, and encouraging the patient to lose weight or change her fluid intake. α-Stimulants or β-blockers are rarely used.

4. The two surgical options for genuine stress incontinence include TVT or colposuspension. Each department has its own favourite between the two. Colposuspension has an 80–90% success rate at 15 years. Anterior repair of the vagina is associated with poor long-term results of 50% continence in 5 years. Sling and Stamey procedures are not appropriate first-line surgical options.

Station 9: Answers

1. Postpartum haemorrhage.

2. Call for HELP! You must not attempt to tackle the patient on your own. You will require the assistance of the Obstetric Registrar, Senior Midwife and Anaesthetist:

   - Insert two large-bore venflons (14 or 16 gauge) for intravenous access and take blood for full blood count, clotting screen, and type and cross 6 units.

   - Take the patient's vital signs.

   - Hang up two bags of gelofusin or Hartmann's solution and run wide open into each intravenous access.

   - Rub the uterus and check the placenta for tears. Check the vagina for tears.

3. Start syntocinon infusion of 40 units in 500 ml normal saline over 4 hours or 40 units in 40 ml normal saline at 10 ml h^{-1} through a syringe driver. Give one ampoule of syntometrine (ergometrine 500 mcg and oxytocin 5 units ml^{-1}) if she is not contracting.

4. If she is hypertensive, do not give syntometrine but rather syntocinon 10 units intramuscularly or intravenously.

5. If bleeding persists and uterine atony is the cause, try carboprost 250 µg intramuscularly. This may be repeated after 20 minutes.

6. If all else fails, consent the patient and take her immediately to theatre for an examination under anaesthesia. Rarely, internal iliac artery ligation or hysterectomy is needed.

Station 10: Answers

1. This is a transvaginal ultrasound scan showing an ectopic pregnancy containing a gestational sac.

2. The incidence for ectopic pregnancies is 1 in 200 pregnancies. Of ectopic pregnancies, 95% occur in the Fallopian tube.

3. Classic symptoms of an ectopic pregnancy include abdominal pain, amenorrhoea and irregular vaginal bleeding. A ruptured ectopic pregnancy will result in shock and peritoneal signs. Referred pain to the shoulder tip may also be present.

4. Predisposing factors to ectopic pregnancy include pelvic inflammatory disease, the use of the IUD, tubal sterilization, *in-vitro* fertilization, GIFT, previous ectopic pregnancy and progestogen-only pills. In other words, if pregnancy occurs, it is more likely to be an ectopic rather than an intrauterine pregnancy.

5. Management of the patient includes resuscitation (gaining intravenous access with two large-bore 14-gauge cannulas and running gelofusin in the lines), taking blood for full blood count and type and cross 4 units, and preparing the patient for theatre for laparoscopic salpingostomy or infusion of methotrexate into the gestational sac. The patient should also be consented for a mini-laparotomy and salpingectomy in case difficulty arises during the laparoscopic approach. Access may be troublesome if there are too many adhesions present, excessive bleeding may warrant an open approach for better control of haemostasis or the ectopic may simply be too large to remove laparoscopically.

Station 11: Answers

1. The surgical instrument is a Kjelland's rotational forceps. (It is also known as Kielland's or Keilland's.) It is characterized by absence of a pelvic curve.

2. This type of forceps is used when rotation of the fetal head is required, i.e. when the occiput is lateral.

3. The eight requirements that must be satisfied for obstetric forceps instrumental delivery include the following:

   - Adequate analgesia (epidural spinal, pudendal or field block).

   - Empty bladder and rectum.

   - No obvious cephalopelvic disproportion.

   - Fully dilated cervix.

   - No head palpable above the pelvic brim.

   - Membranes must not be intact.

   - Position of the fetal head must be known (occipito-anterior, mento-anterior or the after-coming head in a vaginal breech).

   - Head must be at station 2+ or more.

Station 12: Answers

1. The surgical instrument is a Wrigley's forceps.

2. It is used for non-rotational forceps delivery.

3. The indications for forceps delivery include:
   - Poor maternal progress in the second stage caused by either abnormal uterine action or failure of the head to rotate adequately.
   - Maternal disease such as cardiac disease, hypertension, pulmonary disease to avoid strenuous pushing in the second stage.
   - Fetal distress (meconium, signs of fetal hypoxia).
   - To control the after-coming head in a vaginal breech delivery.
   - Following a dural tap at attempted epidural injection.

4. The instrument is a Neville–Barnes forceps.

5. It is used for non-rotational forceps delivery.

1. It is a ventouse cup.

2. The advantages of ventouse delivery over forceps delivery are:
   - Smaller episiotomy.
   - Delivery of occipitotransverse and posterior positions does not require forced rotation of the head.
   - Reduction of the diameter of the presenting part by flexing the head.
   - Less analgesia is required.
   - Less risk of fetal and maternal injury.

3. The potential complications of a ventouse delivery can be divided into maternal and fetal complications:
   - Maternal complications include vaginal wall laceration from entrapment of the vaginal mucosa between the suction cup and fetal head, and risk of cervical damage.
   - Fetal complications include cephalhaematoma, subgaleal haematoma, intracranial haemorrhage and scalp lacerations.

Station 14: Answers

This is a favourite DRCOG OSCE topic.

1. A transvaginal ultrasound image of a uterus containing an intrauterine contraceptive device (IUD, 'a copper coil'). An IUD is clearly distinguishable from an IUS on ultrasound by its distinct borders and increased echogenicity. Compare and contrast this ultrasound image with the one in Circuit A, Station 15.

2. The mode of action of an IUD is to inhibit implantation. The IUD acts before implantation of the blastocyst by stimulating a sterile inflammatory reaction in the endometrium, potentiated by the addition of copper. Additionally, it acts to inhibit sperm migration, fertilization and ovum transport.

3. Absolute contraindications to the use of an IUD include acute and chronic pelvic infection, congenital anomalies of the uterus, copper allergy and Wilson's disease, large fibroids, which distort the uterine cavity, and pregnancy.

4. IUDs can be fitted at any time of the menstrual cycle. They can also be inserted 5 days post-coitally as post-coital contraception or at 8 weeks postpartum. Ensure that the woman is neither pregnant nor has an implanted ovum, as the coil is not an abortifacient!

5. Possible complications associated with the IUD can be divided into early and late complications. Early complications include heavy bleeding, prolonged pain on and after insertion of the coil, and uterine perforation. Late complications include displacement of the IUD, intermenstrual spotting or menorrhagia, pelvic inflammatory disease (anaerobes, actinomycetes, *Chlamydia trachomatis* and *Neisseria gonorrhoea*), partial or complete expulsion of the coil, and pregnancy with an increased relative rate of ectopic pregnancy.

6. The IUD is effective for between 3 and 10 years depending on the individual device. For instance, a first-generation IUD such as Copper T 200 (Ortho Gyne T) is licensed for use in the UK for 3 years. A second-generation IUD such as Nova-T 200 (Novagard) is licensed for use in the UK for up to 5 years. A third-generation IUD such as Copper T Cu 380 A (Gyne 380 Slimline) is licensed for use in the UK for up to 10 years.

This is a favourite DRCOG OSCE topic.

1. The transvaginal ultrasound confirms that the Mirena coil is correctly positioned in the uterine cavity. The ultrasound also shows adenomyosis.

2. Levonorgestrel is the active component, which is released at 20 µg/24 hours. The IUS is a levonorgestrel IUD and consists of a modified Nova-T frame incorporating a silastic capsule on a vertical stem containing 52 mg levonorgestrel.

3. The IUS acts by thickening the cervical mucus, causing endometrial atrophy and partial ovulation suppression.

4. The IUS is associated with a reduction or elimination of menstrual bleeding and has recently been licensed for the treatment of menorrhagia. The IUD is associated with intermenstrual bleeding and menorrhagia. The IUS has also been considered for use in hormone-replacement therapy as a method of opposing oestrogen and protecting the endometrium. Studies suggest a lower rate of PID and a lower relative rate of ectopic pregnancy with the IUS versus the IUD.

5. Disadvantages of the IUS include its prohibitive cost (£100 per device) and the need for local anaesthesia. The diameter of a loaded IUS is 4.8 mm compared with 3.7 mm for a standard Nova-T device. This means dilating the cervical canal to a Hegar 5!

6. The IUS is licensed for use in the UK for up to 5 years.

Station 16: Answers

1. The slide shows a hypha and clue cells. A hypha, or a pseudo-hypha in this case, is a Gram-positive, elongated, budding fungal cell. Clue cells are vaginal epithelial cells covered with many tiny Gram-negative rods. This gives the distinctive 'salt and pepper' appearance.

2. Candidiasis: bacterial vaginosis (*Gardnerella vaginosis*).

3. No, not necessarily. *Candida albicans* appears as Gram-positive oval-budding yeast and Gram-positive, elongated, budding cells resembling hyphae (pseudohyphae). It is a member of the normal vaginal flora.

4. Overgrowth of *Candida* has been associated with diabetes mellitus, immunosuppression, pregnancy and recent antibiotic therapy. *Gardnerella* is a Gram-negative rod and a frequent member of the normal flora of the vagina. Excessive douching or indulging in bubble baths has been associated with the overgrowth of *Gardnerella* and anaerobes, resulting in a frothy, grayish discharge and the distinctive 'fishy' vaginal odour when alkalinized with potassium hydroxide. IUD users are also at increased risk. The pH of the discharge is > 4.6.

5. The treatment for candidiasis (moniliasis) is an antifungal agent such as clotrimazole 500 mg pessary to be inserted at night as a single dose and clotrimazole 1% cream to be applied to the anogenital area two to three times daily. The treatment for BV is oral metronidazole 400 mg bd for 5 days or 2 g as a single dose. The patient should be warned of the disulphiram-like reaction with alcohol.

Station 17: Answers

1. A fetal cardiotocograph.

2. The fetal baseline heart rate is ~150 bpm. The normal baseline heart rate ranges from 110 to 150 bpm. A baseline heart rate > 160 bpm should arouse suspicion. Bear in mind that the baseline rate is higher in preterm babies.

3. The baseline variability is 10 bpm. The normal baseline variability ranges between 10 and 25 bpm.

4. The graph is ominous. The fetal CTG depicts prolonged variable decelerations suggesting fetal distress and compromise. A deceleration is defined as a transient drop in fetal heart rate of at least 15 bpm and lasting for at least 15 seconds. Early decelerations are normal and associated with fetal head compression during a uterine contraction. However, variable decelerations are decelerations that vary in shape, size and timing to contractions and are pathological.

5. An emergency Caesarean section is advisable.

Station 18: Answers

1. The transvaginal ultrasound depicts a 3.2 × 2.7 cm subserous fibroid.

2. There is no cause for alarm. Fibroids are common and benign.

3. Fibroids are located subserous, intramural or submucous.

4. Submucous fibroids are more likely to cause menorrhagia due to their position in the endometrial cavity.

5. Medical treatment includes antifibrinolytic agents such as tranexamic acid (cyklokapron) 1–1.5 g three to four times daily for 3–4 days at the start of each menses, and non-steroidal anti-inflammatory drugs (NSAIDs) such as mefenamic acid 500 mg three times daily prn dysmenorrhoea.

6. Surgical treatment involves myomectomy. The patient should be informed of the small risk of a hysterectomy when consenting to a myomectomy. Zoladex (goserelin) is a gonadorelin analogue. It is administered as a subcutaneous 3.6-mg implant into the anterior abdominal wall every 28 days for 3 months before myomectomy to shrink the fibroid and facilitate surgery. Patients should be warned of the menopause-like symptoms associated with zoladex.

Station 19: Answers

This is a favourite DRCOG OSCE topic.

1. The smear shows a flagellated protozoon or *Trichomonas vaginalis*. The trichomonad is pear-shaped with four anterior flagella and an undulating membrane lined with a flagellum.

2. The organism is isolated on a wet mount smear.

3. *T. vaginalis* thrives in a pH of 5.5–6.0 and can be found in women with an abnormally low vaginal pH (normal 3.8–4.4).

4. *T. vaginalis* may present with raw 'strawberry patches' or petechiae on the cervix and vaginal mucosa.

5. *T. vaginalis* is generally transmitted by sexual intercourse. The patient may complain of a frothy yellow or green rancid vaginal discharge, vaginal and vulvar burning and pruritus, and dyspareunia.

6. The treatment is oral metronidazole 400 mg for 5 days.

7. The patient should be warned of the disulphiram-like reaction of metronidazole when taken with alcohol.

8. The patient should be advised to postpone having sex until both partners are treated or to use a condom. The patient should be advised to return in 2 weeks for a repeat examination and smears/swabs. The patient should be advised to contact her sexual partner and advise him to see his GP or to attend a GUM clinic for testing and treatment.

Station 20: Answers

1. The examination is dark-field or dark-ground microscopy.

2. The organisms shown are spirochetes.

3. This condition is primary syphilis.

4. The specimen was obtained by expressing tissue fluid from a primary syphilitic lesion and placing the drop of fluid or exudate onto a slide with a coverslip. The preparation is then examined under oil immersion with dark-field illumination.

5. The three serologic tests for syphilis are venereal disease research laboratories (VDRL), fluorescent treponemal antibody (FTA) and *Treponema pallidum* haemagglutination (TPHA). VDRL is a low-cost test based on the fact that the particles of the lipid antigen remain dispersed with normal serum but form clumps when combined with reagin. The test reverts to negative in 6–18 months after treatment. FTA uses indirect immunofluorescence (killed *T. pallidum* + patient's serum + labelled antihuman γ-globulin) and has excellent sensitivity and specificity for syphilis antibodies. It is the first test to become positive in early syphilis but remains positive for many years following treatment. TPHA uses red blood cells treated to adsorb treponemes on their surface. The cells clump, if mixed with serum containing antitreponemal antibodies. It is similar in sensitivity and specificity to the FTA test but only becomes positive later in the course of syphilis.

6. According to the *British National Formulary (BNF)*, the treatment of choice for early syphilis is procaine benzylpenicillin (2 ml reconstituted bicillin or 600 mg procaine benzylpenicillin + 120 mg benzylpenicillin sodium) intramuscularly daily for 10–14 days. Alternative treatment is a 14-day course of oral doxycycline (200 mg od) or 14–21 days of oral tetracycline (500 mg qds) or a 14-day course of oral erythromycin (if penicillin-allergic) at 500 mg qds.

7. A Jarisch–Herzheimer reaction may occur within hours after treatment. This is due to the release of toxins from killed spirochetes and immune complex formation. It is a self-limiting febrile condition.

8. The treatment for this reaction is aspirin.

DRCOG OSCE for Circuit B
Answers

Station I: Answers

1. This is an ultrasound depicting spina bifida. Spina bifida is a neural tube defect involving the skin, muscle or bone.

2. The marker for prenatal diagnosis of open neural tube defects is elevated amniotic α-fetoprotein, which results from leakage through exposed vessels. This marker is also raised in other congenital malformations such as omphalocoele and gastroschisis.

3. Spina bifida can be subdivided into spina bifida occulta, meningocele, meningomyelocele and myelocele. Spina bifida occulta is a bone deficit with an intact spinal cord and membranes. Infants may have a hairy tuft or dimple overlying the defect. This deficit carries a good prognosis. Meningocele is a condition in which the neural membranes bulge outwards through a bony deficit. This defect is often small and requires surgical closure. Prognosis is good if there is no associated neurological involvement. Meningomyelocele occurs when the neural plate is exposed or covered with a thin layer of leptomeninges. The exposed lesion should be covered immediately with a sterile non-adhesive dressing. Prognosis depends on the severity of the lesion and of the associated neurological and orthopaedic malformations. Myelocele is defined as exposure of the central cord and is incompatible with life.

4. Problems associated with spina bifida or meningomyelocele, in particular, may include anal and bladder paralysis, chromosomal defects, congenital dislocation of the hips, congenital heart disease, kyphoscoliosis, hydrocephalus, talipes and total paraplegia.

1. Explain to the examiner that you would take a detailed clinical history from the patient. You would wish to know the duration and severity of the PV bleed, any previous bleeding in this pregnancy and if there was any associated abdominal pain, tightenings or uterine contractions. You would also want to know about the fetal movements. Also, if the patient had had recent sexual intercourse. You would inquire as to the date of her last cervical smear and her rhesus status. You are told she is rhesus-negative. You would want to know when her last ultrasound was to confirm her dates and to check the previous position of her placenta to exclude placenta praevia or placental abruptio. You would then ask her about her previous pregnancies and deliveries, and whether she had any underlying medical conditions.

2. On clinical examination, you would palpate the abdomen to assess the site and severity of any abdominal tenderness. You would measure the fundal height and correlate this with the gestation of pregnancy and check the presentation of the fetus. You would also auscultate for fetal heart sounds or use a sonicaid. You would perform a speculum examination to determine the origin of the bleed. You would examine the cervix to exclude cervical polyp, ectropion or erosion. You would **not** perform a digital vaginal examination.

3. Investigations you would arrange for the patient include a urine dipstick, a cardiotocograph to assess for fetal well-being and a transabdominal ultrasound to assess for liquor volume, fetal presentation and well-being, placental localization, and, possibly, to identify the cause of her bleed.

4. You are told that the ultrasound report states that the placenta is in the upper pole, the amniotic fluid volume is normal and the fetus is appropriate for dates. You explain to the examiner that you would reassure the patient and take blood to check her Kleihauer and administer anti-D immunoglobulin according to the level of exposure to rhesus-positive blood in this possibly sensitizing event.

5. Explain that you would document the details of the assessment and treatment in the patient's hand-held notes. Reassure the patient and suggest she return if she has increased PV bleed or abdominal pain.

Station 3: Answers

1. The initial management for the patient is to take a detailed clinical history.

2. On clinical examination, palpate the abdomen to assess for the site and severity of abdominal tenderness and presentation and the position of the fetus. Measure the symphysis-fundal height and correlate it with the gestation of pregnancy or confirm gestation from a recent ultrasound. Perform a PV examination and speculum examination to exclude cervical motion excitation, PV discharge, SROM, or cervical effacement and dilatation.

3. The three investigations you would perform on the patient include a urine dipstick with midstream urine for culture and sensitivity if positive, a full blood count and a transabdominal ultrasound to assess for liquor volume, fetal presentation, placental location and a possible cause for the abdominal pain. (Do not use abbreviations when completing the boxes!)

4. The antibiotic of choice for a UTI in pregnancy is amoxycillin 500 mg o tds for 5 days.

5. If she is penicillin-allergic, trimethoprim 200 mg o bd can be prescribed for 5 days as an alternative.

This is a favourite DRCOG OSCE topic.

1. The diagnosis is primary dysmenorrhoea, which is painful menstruation in the absence of detectable organic or psychological cause. The pain occurs with the onset of menstruation and should then decline.

2. Premenstrual tension may coexist with primary dysmenorrhoea. Symptoms include abdominal bloating, anxiety, breast tenderness, depression, headache and hostility.

3. Treatment for disabling PMT includes a SSRI such as fluoxetine or prescribing cyclic progestogen.

4. The two questions you would ask of the daughter in private are whether she has been sexually abused (psychological component) or whether she is sexually active (organic cause).

5. The medical treatment for primary dysmenorrhoea is mefenamic acid (ponstan) 500 mg o tds for period pains. This prostaglandin synthetase inhibitor will counteract the abnormally high production of endometrial prostaglandins. An alternative treatment would be to offer the girl the combined oral contraceptive (coc) pill if she has no contraindications to its use. If the mother is not aware of her daughter's sexual habits, then the pill should be offered to the daughter in confidence. The pill acts to inhibit ovulation.

Station 5: Answers

1. The maternal blood investigations include Kleihauer, full blood count, electrophoresis, glycosylated haemoglobin, thyroid function tests, TORCH screen and parvovirus.

2. The other maternal investigation to be obtained is a high vaginal swab for microscopy, culture and sensitivity.

3. The placenta should be sent to histology.

4. The options for post-mortem include the following. (1) A full post-mortem, which requires a small sample of each organ for examination and the brain will need to be placed in solution for 5 days before examination. The brain is then returned to the baby. This option also includes removal of fragments of tissue for medical education and research. (2) A full post-mortem but no removal of tissue for medical education and research. (3) A limited post-mortem, which involves a surgical incision and examination of only specified organs. (4) Needle biopsies of organs and no surgical incision. An external examination is conducted, which includes X-rays and medical photographs. The patient should also be offered a fifth option (5), no post-mortem.

Station 6: Answers

This is a favourite DRCOG OSCE topic.

1. The three possible causes for 'wetting' the bed include preterm premature rupture of membranes (PPROM), urinary incontinence and urinary tract infection. The most likely diagnosis is PPROM.

2. Questions you would ask the patient should be focused on excluding or confirming one of your differential diagnoses. If you suspect PPROM, ask if she has any associated contractions. Eighty per cent of PPROM occurrences will initiate labour. If you suspect urinary incontinence, ask her about her prior obstetric history (heavy babies, Caesarean section versus forceps, etc.) and whether she leaks when she coughs or sneezes. The type of urinary incontinence most associated with multiparity is stress incontinence. The mechanism for this form of incontinence is a result of the proximal urethra lying outside the intra-abdominal pressure zone in instances of increased intra-abdominal pressure. Normally, the proximal urethra lies inside the intra-abdominal pressure zone. If you suspect a UTI, ask if she has any associated symptoms of dysuria (burning, frequency or urgency) or suprapubic discomfort.

3. The three things you would perform on clinical examination are a sterile Cusco bivalve speculum examination to confirm PPROM by the presence of liquor (use pH-sensitive nitrazine sticks if unsure), palpation of the abdomen (to assess for fetal lie and presentation and any abdominal tenderness) with CTG monitoring to assess for fetal well-being, and, if you suspected stress incontinence, a Simms speculum examination when asking the patient to cough.

4. The two investigations you would perform would be an endocervical swab for microscopy and culture to exclude group B *Streptococcus* infection, and a urinalysis on a MSU. If the urinalysis is positive for leukocytes, nitrates or protein, send the urine for microscopy, culture and sensitivities.

5. If she has ruptured her membranes, the prognosis is grim at 21 weeks' gestation. The patient should be admitted and covered with intravenous antibiotics. PPROM occurs in up to 40% of all labours. Treatment should be conservative. If intrauterine infection develops, intravenous antibiotics should be administered and labour expedited.

Station 7: Answers

1. The differential diagnosis for severe right-sided lower abdominal pain includes acute appendicitis, acute PID, ectopic pregnancy, complications of an ovarian infection, rupture, torsion or tumour, or acute pyelonephritis. Three likely findings on bimanual, PV and speculum examination include 3+ cervical motion excitation, adnexal tenderness and purulent vaginal discharge.

2. Yes, you would remove the coil as a potential source of infection.

3. The most likely diagnosis is then acute pelvic inflammatory disease.

4. The three investigations you would perform include endocervical swabs for *Chlamydia* (viral form) and gonorrhoea (microbiology form), and a high vaginal swab for *Trichomonas*, *Gardnerella*, candidiasis, etc. (microbiology form); the coil should be sent in a pot for MC&S, and a full blood count obtained to confirm leukocytosis. If in doubt of the diagnosis, a transvaginal ultrasound should be arranged urgently to exclude other causes.

5. According to the *British National Formulary* (*BNF*), the treatment guideline for acute PID is 14 days of metronidazole and doxycycline. The patient should be admitted. She should be prescribed regular analgesia, intravenous metronidazole to cover anaerobic infection and oral doxycycline to cover *Chlamydia* infection. Addition of intravenous amoxycillin, cefotaxime or ciprofloxacin is left to your discretion. Gonorrhoea is treated specifically with a single oral dose of 500 mg ciprofloxacin.

6. Doxycycline is contraindicated in pregnancy. Erythromycin should be substituted. Metronidazole is safe in pregnancy.

Station 8: Answers

This is a favourite DRCOG OSCE topic.

The examiner and the patient (a role-playing actress) will be marking you out of ten possible points, with one point assigned to each of the following points:

1. **Establishing rapport**: introduce yourself to the patient in a friendly manner. Smile, greet her by name and shake her hand.

2. **Verbal/non-verbal cues**: do you pick up cues given by the patient?

3. **Eye contact**: do you maintain good eye contact with the patient?

4. **Take a gynaecological history:**

   - Acknowledge her name and age and ask her why she has come to the clinic. How old were you when your periods started?

   - Age at menarche. When was the first day of your last menstrual period?

   - Do your periods come every 28 or 35 days? Here she may comment that they come irregularly – sometimes skipping a month. Ask her how long they have been irregular.

   - For how many days does the period last? 3–5, 5–7, 7–10, etc.

   - How heavy is the period? Do you pass blood clots? Here she may comment on passage of clots and not being able to leave the house for fear of drenching her outer garments despite wearing sanitary towels.

   - Have you tried any medication for your heavy periods and irregular cycles?

   - Are the periods painful? Does she have a component of dysmenorrhoea?

   - When was your last cervical smear? Have they ever been abnormal or have you ever had colposcopy?

   - What do you use for contraception?

- Have you ever been on the combined oral contraceptive (coc) pill?
- Do you have a regular partner?
- Have you ever had a sexually transmitted disease?
- Do you have any history of gynaecological illnesses such as fibroids, ovarian cysts, etc?
- Do you have any history of gynaecological operations?
- Do you have a family history of cancer of the breast, ovary or womb?

5. **Other relevant history:**
   - Ask her about her obstetric history. How many times has she been pregnant? Has she had any ectopics, TOPs or miscarriages? How many children does she have? What are their ages? What was the mode of delivery (Caesarean elective versus emergency, instrumental or normal vaginal)? Were they term babies? What was the weight of the babies?
   - Ask her briefly about her medical history.
   - Do you suffer from thyroid disease? Hypothyroidism is a cause of menorrhagia.
   - Do you suffer from anaemia?
   - What medicines do you take regularly?
   - Do you have any allergies?

6. **Avoidance of medical jargon.**

7. **Ask the patient if there is anything she would like to add.**

8. **Inform the patient of her options in layman's terms. Reassure the patient.** Explain to her that irregular cycles with heavy bleeding are usual and most likely due to hormonal imbalance. Offer her the option of trying the combined oral contraceptive (coc) pill as a means of both regulating her cycles and diminishing the amount of her bleeds. Explain that you would like to arrange for her a transvaginal ultrasound of the pelvis to exclude the presence of fibroids in her womb. Explain that fibroids are very common and are non-cancerous (benign) muscular outpouchings of the womb that tend to increase bleeding during menstruation.

9. **Ask if she has any further questions and whether she needs anything clarified.**

10. **Would the patient like to see you again?** Offer her a leaflet on the pill and suggest she go away and think about the pill. Offer her a follow-up appointment in a week's time to discuss the pill, and another one to discuss the results of the transvaginal ultrasound in 8 weeks' time.

Station 9: Answers

This is a favourite DRCOG OSCE topic.

The key points to cover are:

1. Explain that you would introduce yourself to the patient and determine why she has chosen to come to you and not the genitourinary medicine (GUM) clinic.

2. Ask her whether she understands what a contact card means and that it only suggests she get tested and that she may not have a sexually transmitted disease. Explain that the GUM clinic cannot release information on which sexually transmitted disease the partner has been treated for.

3. Acknowledge her fears and concerns that there is a stigma attached to attending a GUM clinic.

4. Explain the advantages the GUM clinic has over management by you as the GP.

5. The GUM clinic would provide a better service than you could provide.

6. The GUM clinic would be aware of which particular disease her partner had and, therefore, be more aggressive in checking her over for it.

7. The GUM clinic has an in-house microbiology laboratory and can offer immediate diagnosis of most sexually transmitted diseases so that she can be treated quicker.

8. The GUM clinic stores antibiotics and can administer appropriate antibiotics free of charge. As she is pregnant, alternative antibiotics would be offered to her that would not affect the fetus.

9. The GUM clinic is anonymous so that your GP may not be privy to her results. As a GP, you may be obliged to inform insurance companies if she has undergone HIV testing, for instance.

10. Explain to her the implications of not getting treated properly – the risks to herself of pelvic inflammatory disease and future infertility and the risks to her unborn child of blindness or fetal abnormalities.

11. Explain to the examiner that the cost implications for the NHS are enormous if she does not get treated and she risks complications for herself and risks passing on the disease to others. The examiner will be delighted that you are aware of the growing costs of NHS healthcare and the need to access healthcare in the most cost efficient way.

Station 10: Answers

This is a favourite DRCOG OSCE topic.

1. **Establish rapport.** Introduce yourself to the patient in a friendly manner and ask her how you can help her?

2. **Verbal/non-verbal cues.** Notice whether she is anxious or deeply concerned. Give her a nod that you acknowledge her concerns. Ask her if she is concerned that she may not be able to conceive?

3. **Maintain eye contact.** Keep your eyes on the patient. Listen sympathetically.

4. **Determine her risks of infertility:**
   - Ask her if her periods are regular?
   - Ask her if she has ever been treated for a sexually transmitted disease or pelvic inflammatory disease.
   - Ask her if she or her partner have any chronic medical ailments?
   - Ask her if she is taking any medication and if so, which ones?
   - Ask her if she has had any operations that might interfere with her ability to conceive?
   - Ask her if she or her partner have any family history of congenital abnormalities?

5. **Offer her general preconception advice:**
   - Suggest that she and her partner limit alcohol intake, stop smoking, eat a healthy diet and take up exercise.
   - Suggest she have frequent intercourse especially around the time of ovulation. Ovulation usually occurs 2 weeks before the onset of menstruation.
   - Suggest she take folic acid supplements when she first notices she is pregnant.

6. **Avoid medical jargon.**

7. **Reassure her.** Explain that you see no reason why she should have any difficulty in conceiving and that 80% of active couples will conceive within 1 year.

8. **Ask her if she has any further questions or needs any points clarified.**

9. **Suggest she make a follow-up appointment.** She should see you as soon as she realizes she is pregnant so that you can offer her immediate antenatal care and take the necessary antenatal bloods.

10. **Does the patient wish to see you again?** The role-playing actress has the option to give this point.

Station 11: Answers

This is a favourite DRCOG OSCE topic.

1. Three possible diagnoses include high suspicion of ectopic pregnancy, threatened miscarriage or ruptured corpus luteum cyst.

2. This patient will require an urgent transvaginal ultrasound to determine whether she has an ectopic pregnancy or a viable intrauterine pregnancy.

3. The two blood tests you would arrange are for hCG and progesterone levels (both can be taken in the same clotted blood tube).

4. King's College Hospital Guidelines for Pregnancy of Unknown Location are as follows:

Progesterone (nmol l^{-1})	hCG (IU l^{-1})	Likely diagnosis	Follow-up
< 20	> 20	failing pregnancy	hCG in 1 week
20–60	> 20	high risk of ectopic	hCG in 48 hours
> 60	< 1000	normal pregnancy	U/S when expected, hCG > 1000 IU l^{-1}
> 60	> 1000	ectopic pregnancy	laparoscopy

5. With pregnancies that cannot be localized on transvaginal ultrasound and high pregnancy hormones, a laparoscopy is mandatory.

6. The three treatments for ectopic pregnancy include conservative management by following the pregnancy with serial transvaginal ultrasounds and serial hCG and progesterone levels, injection of the ectopic with methotrexate under ultrasonic guidance, and laparoscopic salpingotomy or salpingectomy. Conservative management is only advisable if hCG < 1000 IU l^{-1}, and there is no visible fetal heart beat. Tubal abortion may occur spontaneously. If this does not occur, the patient will need an urgent laparoscopy. The patient should be warned of the risk of a mini-laparotomy if difficulty arises using the laparoscopic approach.

7. This patient requires anti-D immunoglobulin. Threatened miscarriages require anti-D prophylaxis at any gestation. The King's College Hospital guidelines = 500 IU anti-D.

Station 12: Answers

1. The most likely diagnosis is gonorrhoea. Men often present with copious yellow-green pus from the urethra and women with a yellow-green vaginal discharge that streams out of the cervix and vagina.

2. Gonorrhoea may be associated with Bartholin's abscess, acute salpingitis and PID.

3. Another possibility for yellow-green vaginal discharge is *Trichomonas vaginalis*, a flagellated protozoon infection. This infection is irritative and produces a frothy discharge.

4. Swabs for GC may be taken from the oral cavity (pharynx), endocervix, urethra and anus. Ask the patient which type of intercourse she has had.

5. Yes, gonorrhoea is seen as Gram-negative diplococci.

6. The standard treatment of a single dose of 500 mg ciprofloxacin is contraindicated in pregnancy. According to the Caldecot Centre GUM Clinic Guidelines for treatment of GC in a pregnant woman, 3 g amoxycillin is offered instead. This can be administered in powdered form mixed in a flavoured drink.

Station 13: Answers

The examiner and the patient (a role-playing actress) will be marking you out of ten possible points, with one point assigned to each of the following points:

1. **Establishing rapport.** Introduce yourself to the patient in a friendly manner. Smile, greet her by name and shake her hand.

2. **Verbal/non-verbal cues.** Do you notice cues of anxiety given off by the patient and allay her concerns?

3. **Eye contact.** Do you maintain good eye contact with the patient?

4. **Explain the results – the following suggestions are obtained from *Cervical Smear Results Explained*, a booklet guide for primary care published by the NHS Cervical Screening Programme.** Explain to the patient that her cervical smear has shown some abnormalities. Explain that 1 in 12 women have abnormal smears that require further investigation with colposcopy. Explain that it is very rare for these abnormalities to be cancerous. Explain that some of these abnormalities will return to normal on their own and most can be cured after a simple, outpatient procedure. Explain that severe dyskaryosis may reflect the presence of cervical intraepithelial neoplasia (CIN), changes which are invisible on inspection by the naked eye and do not harm the patient at present, but if left untreated, there is a risk of progressing to invasive cancer.

5. **Explain the procedure of colposcopy.** Explain that the procedure is performed in the Outpatient Clinic by a Gynaecologist, and no anaesthetic is required. Explain that the procedure only takes 10–15 minutes. Explain that she will be lying on a couch with her legs in leg rests very similar to when she had the smear taken. A speculum will be inserted, and the cervix is brought into view under the magnifying colposcope. The instrument is positioned between her legs but does not enter her. The cervix is examined. A smear may be retaken. Acetic acid solution is applied to any abnormal areas and may sting slightly. An iodine solution may be applied to reveal the outer limits of any abnormal areas. A biopsy may also be taken to aid in diagnosis and the sampling may be

slightly uncomfortable. She will be informed of the diagnosis and may be offered appropriate treatment at the same appointment.

6. **Avoid medical jargon.**

7. **Ask the patient if she has understood your explanation and whether she has any questions.** She asks you to explain what the treatment is for an abnormal cervix? Will she end up having a hysterectomy? Explain to her that no, she will not require a hysterectomy. Explain that the present methods of treatment of CIN are aimed to remove or destroy any abnormal cells (found in the transformation zone of the cervix). This is done using local anaesthesia. Treatment options include local destructive therapy with a carbon dioxide laser, 'cold' coagulation, cryosurgery or electrocoagulation. In other words, treatment is by extremes of cold or heat. The abnormal area may also be locally excised by knife cone biopsy, laser cone biopsy or large loop excision of the transformation zone (LLETZ). Explain that she may experience cramp-like pain (uterine contractions), and that cervical function is not affected.

8. **Reassure the patient.**

9. **Discuss follow-up.** Inform the patient that she will need a repeat colposcopy appointment in 6 months to reassure both herself and the Gynaecologist that there is no residual disease or new findings.

10. **Would the patient like to see you again?** Have you conducted yourself in a polite, caring, fluent and professional manner?

Station 14: Answers

1. The four investigations you should perform in the clinic are bimanual and speculum examination (to assess for a fibroid uterus or the presence of a cervical polyp or ectropion), endo-cervical and high vaginal swabs (to exclude an infective cause), a cervical smear test (to exclude neoplasia) and a full blood count (to exclude anaemia).

2. You should refer the patient for a transvaginal ultrasound to be performed on the last day of her period when the endometrial lining is thin to allow for assessment of an endometrial polyp. The lining of the endometrium thickens thereafter and will obscure ultrasound interpretation. The uterus can also be assessed for the presence of fibroids and whether the fibroids are distorting the lining of the endometrial cavity. This is important when considering IUCD or IUS insertion.

3. This patient is not suitable for the combined oral contraceptive (coc) pill as she is a smoker > 35 years of age.

4. Her choices for contraception that will also manage her bleed-ing include the IUS (Mirena), which has now been licensed for the management of menorrhagia, contraceptive injectables and the progestogen-only pill. The patient should be warned that the IUS may be associated with irregular light bleeding for the first 3 months. The latter two are not as favourable as she is already 90 kg in weight and may not wish to risk further weight gain. The progestogen-only pill will need to be taken in double the dose as she weighs > 70 kg.

5. Her surgical options include hysterectomy or endometrial ablation.

Station 15: Answers

This is a favourite DRCOG OSCE topic.

1. FSH > 30 IU l⁻¹ and oestradiol < 70 pmol l⁻¹ are diagnostic of menopause.

2. Symptoms associated with the menopause include vasomotor symptoms (hot flushes, palpitations, dizziness, night sweats), psychological symptoms (depression, anxiety, irritability, poor memory, poor concentration), symptoms due to urogenital atrophy (superficial dyspareunia secondary to vaginal dryness, loss of libido, urinary frequency, urge incontinence), and signs of skin changes (thin, dry skin, brittle nails, hair loss). The patient is at long-term risk of osteoporosis and cardiovascular disease.

3. Three forms of treatment include combined oestrogen–progesterone HRT, tibolone (a synthetic steroid with weak oestrogenic, progestogenic and androgenic effects), and selective oestrogen receptor modulators. Unopposed oestrogen therapy places the patient at risk for endometrial carcinoma. The addition of progesterone removes the excess risk but brings about monthly withdrawal bleeds. Tibolone (Livial) is recommended for menopausal patients with loss of libido due to its androgenic effect. It is a 'no period' preparation. Selective (o)estrogen receptor modulators (SERMs) such as raloxifene have a beneficial effect on both lipid profiles and vertebral osteoporosis, but not on the vasomotor symptoms associated with menopause. It does not stimulate the endometrium and may reduce the risk of breast cancer. It is not recommended for women with vasomotor symptoms.

4. If the patient has had a hysterectomy, she can be offered oestrogen therapy alone without the addition of progesterone as she has no endometrial lining to protect. Routes of oestrogen therapy administration include oral, transdermal, subcutaneous, vaginal, sublingual or intranasal.

Station 16: Answers

1. Breast-feeding protects the baby against ear infections, chest infections, diarrhoea, gastroenteritis and eczema. The baby has better mouth formation with straighter teeth and less smelly nappies.

2. Breast-feeding for the mother protects her against ovarian cancer and premenopausal breast cancer. She has a faster return to a prepregnancy state. Breast-feeding can also be used as a form of natural contraception for the first 6 months.

3. The three conditions that must be met to use the lactational amenorrhoea method of contraception include no menses, no supplemental feeds other than breast-feeding and the baby must be < 6 months of age.

4. The risk of pregnancy using the lactational amenorrhoea method is 1–2%. The mother should be advised of alternative forms of postpartum contraception if she wishes the risk to be nil. The progestogen-only pill is safely administered from 6 weeks postpartum in women who breast-feed. The combined oral contraceptive (coc) pill is contraindicated in breast-feeding women as the oestrogen component inhibits the production of breast milk. An alternative form of contraception is the Levonorgestrel-releasing intrauterine system (LNG-IUS), which may be inserted at 6 weeks postpartum in breast-feeding women. The delay in insertion is to avoid the high expulsion rates associated with post-placental insertion. Female sterilization may also be offered but is not recommended at the time of Caesarean section due to higher failure rates associated with oedematous, vascular Fallopian tubes and a higher incidence of regret.

Station 17: Answers

1. Causes of preterm labour include idiopathic (50%), antepartum haemorrhage, cervical incompetence, maternal pyrexia, multiple pregnancy, polyhydramnios, preterm premature rupture of the membranes, pyelonephritis, fetal death and uterine abnormalities.

2. Management of preterm labour involves attempting to establish a cause for it. Perform an abdominal to assess for abdominal tenderness and fetal presentation, and a speculum examination to assess whether the membranes are intact and to take high vaginal swabs for microscopy, culture and sensitivities. If the membranes are intact, perform a PV exam to assess for cervical length and dilatation, the station and nature of the presenting part. Urinalysis should be performed on a midstream urine sample to exclude infection. The patient should be attached to a CTG monitor to assess for fetal well-being.

3. If the cervix is < 4 cm dilated, tocolytic agents have been shown to delay delivery for 72 hours. GTN patches (10 mg) should be applied topically to the abdomen for gestations up to 34 weeks. Steroid therapy (dexamethasone 12 mg intravenously) should also be administered to reduce the incidence of death from respiratory distress syndrome (RDS) between the gestations of 28 and 32 weeks.

Station 18: Answers

1. The gynaecological causes of chronic pelvic pain include pelvic pain syndrome, endometriosis, chronic pelvic inflammatory disease, pelvic adhesions, ovarian remnant syndrome, IUCD use and dysmenorrhoea. The most likely diagnosis for the patient is pelvic pain syndrome or pelvic vein congestion. Typically, the pain alternates between aching and being sharp in nature and is worse on standing, after exercise, during the second half of the menses or after a bowel movement. This is in contrast to irritable bowel syndrome, where the pain is relieved by opening of the bowels. The patient may also complain of a post-coital ache. The pain is eased by lying down and by applying heat or a hot-water bottle to the lower abdomen. One explanation for this syndrome is pelvic vein congestion as demonstrated on pelvic venography by the pooling of contrast in the pelvic veins with dilatation of the pelvic veins to 10–15 mm from 3 mm.

2. Endocervical and high vaginal swabs should be taken in clinic to exclude PID.

3. The three investigations you should arrange for the patient include a transvaginal ultrasound, pelvic venography and laparoscopy.

4. According to Mr A. Davies' Chronic Pelvic Pain Clinic, King's College Hospital, the three forms of treatment for pelvic pain syndrome include counselling and reassurance, a 6-month course of Provera (medroxyprogesterone acetate) 10 mg o tds or a GnRH agonist ± add-back therapy, or TAH/BSO as a last resort.

1. The most likely diagnosis is endometriosis. Endometriosis may be associated with obesity, short menstrual cycles of long duration, uterine retroversion, secondary dysmenorrhoea, dyspareunia, chronic pelvic pain, dyschesia (pain on opening the bowels) and infertility. Physical findings may include nodules along the uterosacral ligament, fixed, retroverted uterus, nodules in surgical scars, cervical motion tenderness or pelvic tenderness.

2. Investigations include pelvic ultrasound, which may demonstrate a ground glass appearance, serum immunoassay of CA-125, and laparoscopy with biopsy. CA-125 > 1000 IU suggests carcinoma, but CA-125 in the low 100s suggests endometriosis. CA-125 increases in response to peritoneal lining irritation.

3. Medical treatment for endometriosis includes the combined oral contraceptive (coc) pill (taken three packets a time with a week's gap), progestogens (Provera) to induce a pseudo-pregnant state, danazol, gestrinone, GnRH agonists such as zoladex injections ± add-back therapy, and the Mirena IUS (experimental). Patients on danazol must be warned of the potential androgenic and anti-oestrogenic side-effects such as greasy hair, acne, irreversible voice deepening, hot flushes, etc. Therapy is discontinued after 6 months to reduce the risk of osteoporosis. Patients on zoladex should be warned of vasomotor side-effects. Therapy is discontinued after 6 months to reduce the risk of osteoporosis.

4. Surgical treatment for endometriosis includes diathermy, excision or laser vaporization of the endometrial deposits, ovarian cystostomy for endometrioma with removal of the lining of the cyst by diathermy to prevent reoccurrence, presacral neurectomy/LUNA, or hysterectomy/BSO (to remove cyclical oestrogen that could stimulate peritoneal endometriosis) + HRT (to prevent osteoporosis).

Station 20: Answers

1. Sperm volume < 2 ml is called aspermia. Sperm density < 20 million ml^{-1} is called oligozoospermia (low count). Sperm motility < 50% progressively motile is called asthenozoospermia (low motility). Sperm morphology < 30% normal shapes is called teratozoospermia (low proportion to normal shape).

2. Other investigations for male infertility include FSH level and size of testes, screening for haemoglobinopathies, LH/FSH and testosterone, karyotype and cystic fibrosis screen if azoospermic, and testicular biopsy. If azoospermic, distinguish between obstructive and non-obstructive aetiology. A high FSH and small testes suggest end-organ failure. A low FSH and small testes suggest pituitary-level failure. A normal FSH and normal size testes suggest obstruction.

3. Options available to the couple are IVF (*in-vitro* fertilization), IUI (intrauterine insemination), ICSI (single intracytoplasmic sperm injection into each oocyte), and DI (donor insemination). ICSI offers a higher pregnancy rate than IVF with a live birth rate of 28% per cycle. In cases of azoospermia, sperm retrieval directly from the testes and epididymis in combination with ICSI or, alternatively, donor insemination can be offered.

DRCOG OSCE for Circuit C Answers

Station 1: Answers

1. You suspect SROM with meconium-stained liquor. You should advise her to come to labour ward immediately.

2. You decide to admit the patient for induction of labour.

3. To induce labour in an unfavourable cervix, administer 1 mg prostin (2 mg in a primip). Repeat in 6 hours if required.

4. Fresh meconium in the liquor may be associated with neonatal hypoxia, umbilical cord compression, uterine hypertonicity, intrauterine growth retardation (IUGR) or post-dates.

5. The CTG suggests umbilical cord compression. A fetal scalp pH may be performed but, ultimately, the patient requires emergency Caesarean section for fetal distress.

6. Potential complications associated with a Caesarean section should be hand-written in the consent form and include bleeding, infection, bladder or bowel injury, and placenta accreta.

This is a favourite DRCOG OSCE topic.

1. You suspect puerperal depression. This condition may present up to 3 months after delivery and occurs in up to 25% of births. Puerperal depression may present with symptoms of anxiety, guilt, depression and conflict with caring for the baby. In contrast, puerperal baby-blues is short-lived and presents 3–5 days after delivery. It is associated with tearfulness and depression and is quite common, occurring in up to 50% of births. It has a good prognosis with reassurance, counselling and night sedation or analgesia, if required. Factors that prolong baby-blues and may contribute to the development of depression include inadequate sleep, delay in healing of a C-section scar or episiotomy (painful perineum), tender breast engorgement, traumatic delivery, prolonged labour, puerperal pyrexia, anaemia and lack of social contacts.

2. Factors associated with puerperal depression include stressful pregnancy or traumatic delivery, lack of social support, being > 30 years of age, lack of sleep, prior history of mood disorders or pre-existing depression and prolonged breast-feeding.

3. Puerperal psychosis usually presents from day 7 and occurs in 1 in 500 births. Clinical manifestations include mania, schizophrenia, suicidal tendencies and/or severe depression. Severe depression is distinguished from mild depression by: psychomotor retardation, early morning awakening, loss of appetite, anhedonia, inability to concentrate and ideas of worthlessness.

4. The recommended treatment for puerperal psychosis includes antipsychotics and antidepressants (SSRIs).

5. The management of puerperal psychosis requires admission for both the mother and, if possible, the baby under the Psychiatrist's care. Puerperal depression in the absence of psychotic delusions may be managed as an outpatient with antidepressant therapy.

Station 3: Answers

This is a favourite DRCOG OSCE topic.

1. Causes of postmenopausal bleeding include endometrial carcinoma (unless proven otherwise), cervical or vulval carcinoma, cervical or endometrial polyp, atrophic vaginitis, oestrogen withdrawal, or infection with *Trichomonas* or candidiasis if associated with post-coital bleeding.

2. In Casualty, ensure that the patient is haemodynamically stable. Take a full history. Examine the vulva and vagina. Perform a speculum examination to exclude cervical polyp or ectropion. Take high vaginal and endocervical swabs to exclude infection. Take a cervical smear to exclude cervical carcinoma. Take blood for full blood count and group and save.

3. Arrange for an urgent transvaginal ultrasound ± pipelle endometrial biopsy and follow-up in the outpatient gynaecology clinic to arrange for hysteroscopy and biopsy.

Station 4: Answers

This is a favourite DRCOG OSCE topic.

1. The test used to confirm diabetes is the 75 g oral glucose tolerance test (OGTT).

2. The patient's insulin requirements will rise during her pregnancy and fall throughout labour. Requirements return to prepregnancy levels a day after delivery. Insulin resistance in pregnancy is due to the placental secretion of oestrogen, progestogen and human placental lactogen, and a change in peripheral insulin receptors.

3. Maternal complications associated with diabetic pregnancy include aggravation of proliferative diabetic retinopathy, pre-eclampsia in mothers with diabetic nephropathy, an increase in first and second trimester miscarriages, preterm labour, polyhydramnios, and sudden intrauterine death in the last 4 weeks of pregnancy.

4. Fetal complications associated with diabetic pregnancy include macrosomia, shoulder dystocia, respiratory distress syndrome (RDS), hypoglycaemia, hypothermia, hypercalcaemia, polycythaemia (hyperbilirubinaemia), congenital malformations (sacral agenesis) and intrauterine death.

5. Plan to deliver the baby vaginally at 38–40 weeks' gestation. If labour is prolonged, proceed to a Caesarean section.

Station 5: Answers

1. The most likely diagnosis is polycystic ovarian syndrome or Stein–Leventhal syndrome (named after Stein and Leventhal in 1935). The hormone profile shows an LH/FSH ratio = 3:1, with an elevated testosterone level. The SHBG level will be low. PCO is a syndrome of unknown aetiology characterized by ovarian, hypothalamic–pituitary and adrenal dysfunction. These patients suffer from hyperinsulinaemia, which leads to weight gain and increased ovarian androgen production. Hepatic synthesis of SHBG is inhibited.

2. Symptoms and signs associated with this syndrome include acne, amenorrhoea or oligomenorrhoea, hirsutism, hyper-insulinaemia, infertility, recurrent miscarriages (RM) and weight gain.

3. The investigation used to confirm PCO is a transvaginal ultra-sound to demonstrate characteristic polycystic ovaries (enlarged with a peripheral ring of follicles).

4. Medical treatment for PCO in those who wish to conceive involves induction therapy with clomiphene and then gonadorelin (gonadotrophin-releasing hormone).

5. If the patient does not wish to conceive, she may be started on the combined oral contraceptive (coc) pill, i.e. Dianette, which contains ethinyl oestradiol and cyproterone acetate (a potent anti-androgen). The latter component will control both the acne and hirsutism.

6. Two surgical treatments for PCO include wedge resection of the ovaries, or laparoscopic laser or diathermy to the ovaries. The latter involves drilling multiple holes in the ovaries to destroy the androgen-producing stroma. This treatment enhances ovulation rates.

Station 6: Answers

The examiner and the patient (a role-playing actress) will be marking you out of ten possible points, with one point assigned to each of the following points:

Remember the mnemonic for counselling: GATHER!

1. **Establishing rapport. Greet** the patient and introduce yourself in a friendly manner. Smile, greet her by name and shake her hand.

2. **Verbal/non-verbal cues.** Do you notice cues given by the patient?

3. **Eye contact.** Do you maintain good eye contact with the patient?

4. **Ask** the patient what her understanding about hormonal contraception is.

5. **Tell** the patient about her options. Explain that the choices for hormonal contraception include the combined oral contraceptive (coc) pill, progestogen-only pill, contraceptive injection, progestogen implant, Mirena IUS (intrauterine system) and the IUD (intrauterine device).

6. **Help** her decide:

   - Explain that the coc pill is > 99% effective.
   - Explain that the coc works by inhibiting ovulation (stopping the release of an egg each month). Explain that the advantages of the coc are that it reduces period pain and bleeding and protects against cancer of the ovary and womb.
   - Explain that the progestogen-only pill is 99% effective and is a once-a-day pill but must be taken at the same time every day and is not effective if > 3 hours late.
   - Explain that this pill is suitable for smokers > 35 years of age and can be used during breast-feeding.
   - Explain that the contraceptive injection (Depo-Provera) is > 99% effective and lasts for 12 weeks and that Noristerat lasts for 8 weeks.

- Explain that the implant lasts for 3 years and is inserted under the skin of the inner upper arm under local anaesthesia.
- Explain that for both the injections and the implant, she may have irregular periods for up to a year and may gain weight.
- Explain that the IUS is >99% effective and works for 5 years.
- Explain that the IUD is 98–99% effective and works for up to 10 years depending on the type used. The IUD is not recommended for women with heavy and painful periods or those with multiple partners. She states she would like to be started on the coc pill.

7. • **Explain** to her that she should have no absolute contra-indications to use of the pill such as heart or liver disease, hypertension, migraine with focal aura, breast cancer, unexplained vaginal bleeding, etc.
- Explain that the pill (e.g. Microgynon) is started on day 1 of her menstrual cycle and that it is recommended that one uses a condom for the first week.
- Explain that she will bleed for 7 days between days 21 and 28.
- Explain that if she misses a pill and it has been over 12 hours, she should take two pills and use a condom for the next 7 days.
- Explain that if she misses four pills, she must go back 1 day only in the pack and use a condom for the next 7 days.
- Explain that if there are seven or more pills left in her pack after the missed pill, she should leave the usual 7-day break when she finishes the pack before starting the next pack.
- Explain that if there are less than seven pills left in the pack after the missed pill, she should start the next pack the next day when she finishes the pack. She must not have the usual 7-day break.
- Explain that she may experience temporary side-effects depending on her hormonal levels. Reported side-effects include a headache, nausea, breast tenderness, bleeding between periods and mood changes.
- Explain that the pill is less effective if she suffers from vomiting or diarrhoea.

- Explain that she can obtain emergency contraception if she is concerned that her method has failed.

8. **Return.** Explain that you would take a complete history and check her height, weight and blood pressure. As long as she did not have any contraindications, you would offer her Microgynon. Also, offer her a contraceptive pamphlet to take home. Suggest she make a follow-up appointment. She may think of other questions to ask you, and you can obtain feedback on how she is managing with the pill.

Station 7: Answers

1. The diagnosis is pre-eclampsia. This condition presents after 20 weeks' gestation. Risk factors include primiparity, height < 155 cm, age < 20 or > 35 years, family history of pre-eclampsia and a history of migraines or renal disease. Smoking is protective!

2. Associated symptoms and signs of pre-eclampsia include chest or epigastric pain, frontal and occipital headache, visual disturbances, fever, vomiting, a rapid rise in blood pressure or a rise of > 30/20 mmHg over the booking BP, hyper-reflexia and clonus.

3. The patient should be admitted that day and her blood pressure rechecked in 4 hours.

4. Investigations should include blood tests (full blood count, clotting screen, urea and electrolytes, liver function tests, group and save), midstream urine for microscopy, culture and sensitivities, 24-hour urine collection for protein, fetal cardio-tocograph, biophysical profile and transabdominal ultrasound to check on the well-being of the fetus.

5. Intravenous hydralazine or labetalol should be administered to control maternal blood pressure. The aim is to control the blood pressure, prevent eclamptic fits and expedite delivery of the baby.

This is a favourite DRCOG OSCE topic.

1. The Pearl Index was named after Dr Raymond Pearl in 1932 and represents the number of pregnancies observed in a cohort of women using a given method divided by the total number of cycles in which the method was used by all the women added together. This number is then multiplied by 1300 to standardize the results to reflect the experience of 100 woman-years with each woman contributing 13 cycles per year. Simply put, the Pearl Index is the failure rate per 100 woman-years of any given contraceptive method.

2. The Pearl Index or the failure rate per 100 woman-years (HWY) = total number of pregnancies × 1300/total months of use for all those using method.

3. The Pearl Index for male or female sterilization is quoted as < 1 per HWY.

4. The Pearl Index for the progestogen-only pill is quoted as 2–3 per HWY.

5. The Pearl Index for the combined oral contraceptive is quoted as < 1 per HWY.

6. The Pearl Index for the Depo-Provera injection is quoted as < 1 per HWY.

7. The Pearl Index for the IUS (Mirena) is quoted as < 1 per HWY.

8. The Pearl Index for the IUCD used to be 2–3 per HWY. However, the new, improved IUDs contain more copper (Multiload Cu 375 and Ortho-Gynae T Cu 380 A) and have a Pearl Index of < 1 per HWY.

9. The Pearl Index for the lactational amenorrhoea method is quoted as 2–3 per HWY.

10. The Pearl Index for the cervical cap with spermicide is quoted recently as high as 8–20 per HWY due to user failure and accidental dislodgement of the cap during intercourse. The Pearl Index for the diaphragm with spermicide is quoted as 4–8 per HWY. The Pearl Index for the condom with spermicide is published as anywhere from 3 to 23 per HWY.

Station 9: Answers

This is a favourite DRCOG OSCE topic.

The examiner and the patient (a role-playing actress) will be marking you out of ten possible points, with one point assigned to each of the following points:

Remember the mnemonic for counselling: GATHER!

1. **Establishing rapport. Greet** the patient by name and introduce yourself in a friendly manner, shaking the patient's hand.

2. **Verbal/non-verbal cues.** Do you notice cues of anxiety given by the patient?

3. **Eye contact.** Do you maintain good eye contact with the patient?

4. **Avoid medical jargon.** Keep your language simple.

5. **Ask** the patient an open-ended question to initiate the discussion.

6. **Tell** the patient that her risk of carrying a Down's syndrome baby is only 1 in 109 at 40 years of age and that the overall incidence of Down's syndrome is 1 in 650 live births.

7. **Help** the patient understand. **Explain** that there are two screening tests for Down's syndrome, namely the nuchal translucency test which is an ultrasound scan to measure the baby's skin for thickness performed at 11–12 weeks and the Bart's triple blood test for oestriol, α-fetoprotein and β-hCG performed at 14–16 weeks' gestation. These tests give 'risks' for carrying a Down's baby but no definite answers. The two diagnostic tests for Down's syndrome include chorionic villus sampling (CVS), which is performed after 9 weeks' gestation, and amniocentesis, which is performed at 16 weeks. CVS involves obtaining fetal tissue from the chorion, the edge of the placenta, using a plastic cannula under ultrasound guidance. The risks of CVS include a 2–4% fetal loss rate, bleeding, perforation of the amniotic sac and infection. The advantage is that the results can be obtained within 48 hours. The fetal tissue is sent for DNA analysis and gene probing. Full cultures take ~2–3 weeks.

Amniocentesis is performed at 16 weeks' gestation and has a lower abortion rate (< 1%), but the results take longer to come back (up to 3 weeks). Ask the patient if she has any questions.

8. **Return.** Offer to refer the patient for CVS and to see her again for follow-up.

Station 10: Answers

Maintain good eye contact with the examiner and answer the questions clearly. Offer the examiner your candidate number and the scoring sheet from your pack of numbered station sheets. Take a seat. The examiner will then ask you if you are ready.

1. Begin by addressing the first topic – the pros of HRT. Explain that the advantages may be divided into short- and long-term benefits. Explain that the short-term benefits include relief of vasomotor symptoms (flushing, palpitations, dizziness, weakness/faintness), relief of the psychological symptoms of menopause (poor memory and concentration, emotional lability, depressed mood), relief of vaginal and bladder symptoms due to urogenital atrophy, and increased moisture to the skin. Explain that with the menopause there is generalized loss of collagen from the dermal layer of the skin, leading to dry skin and widespread joint and muscle aches. Explain that the long-term benefits of HRT include protection against osteoporosis after 5 years of HRT with a 50% reduction in hip fractures, a 40% reduction in the risk of coronary artery disease and slowing of the progression of Alzheimer's disease.

2. Explain that the cons of HRT may be divided into short- and long-term side-effects. The short-term side-effects include those due to oestrogen (breast tenderness, headache, leg cramps), which only last a few months, and those due to progesterone (bloating, weight gain, mood swings) seen in 5% of patients, and irregular vaginal bleeding. The long-term side-effects include increased risk of breast cancer after 10 years (with no change in mortality rate of breast cancer in HRT users and non-users), a 3–5-fold increased risk of endometrial carcinoma with unopposed oestrogen, and a 2-fold increase in the risk of deep venous thrombosis (DVT) in the first year of use.

3. Explain that the HRT may be offered in the form of creams, implants, injections, nasal spray, transdermal patches, pessaries or tablets. Explain that the different forms of HRT include systemic sequential combined HRT, continuous combined HRT, unopposed oestrogen (post-hysterectomy), progestogen-only therapy, gonadomimetic (tibolone) and selective (o)estrogen receptor modulators (SERMs). Tibolone has oestrogenic, progestogenic and androgenic effects and treats menopausal symptoms and protects against osteoporosis. It is a

no-bleed HRT for use in women at least 1 year postmenopause. SERMs, i.e. raloxifene, are licensed for the prevention and treatment of spinal osteoporosis and also have an oestrogen-like effect on bones and the vagina, with an anti-oestrogen effect on the breasts and endometrium. Explain that local HRT is offered as oestrogen only.

4. Explain that as the cost implications of treating osteoporotic-related fractures are high, with both one in four women in their 60s and one in two women in their 70s suffering from an osteoporotic-related fracture, the use of HRT should be encouraged. Explain that the cost-effectiveness of HRT is unknown as many postmenopausal women choose not to 'interfere' with nature.

Station 11: Answers

This is a favourite DRCOG OSCE topic.

1. Initial tests used to investigate prolonged neonatal jaundice (jaundice lasting > 14 days) include serum total and direct bilirubin levels, serum liver function tests, full blood count and film, full infection screen, and thyroid function tests. An abdominal ultrasound scan, colloid liver scanning and biopsy are second-line investigations.

2. The causes of prolonged neonatal jaundice include breast milk jaundice (most common cause), congenital infection (TORCH – toxoplasmosis, rubella, CMV, *Herpes* or hepatitis A, B or C), endocrine disorders (hypopituitarism, congenital hypothyroidism), extrahepatic biliary atresia, genetic disorders (cystic fibrosis and α-1-antitrypsin deficiency), inborn errors of metabolism (galactosaemia, tyrosinaemia), and intrahepatic biliary hypoplasia. The colour of the motions should be checked. Pale stools and dark urine are associated with conjugated hyperbilirubinaemia. Breast milk jaundice is associated with unconjugated hyperbilirubinaemia.

1. She is not a suitable candidate as she has health risks. She has a high BMI and is, therefore, at risk if she undergoes general anaesthesia. In particular, she is at risk from a pulmonary embolism. Her new partner needs to be tested first to exclude male infertility. There are cost implications that need to be considered with regards to NHS resources.

2. Suggestions you would offer would be for her to lose weight, arrange for a seminal fluid analysis from her new partner, wait to see how long this current relationship will last, and ask herself what her motives are. Does she want a baby to cement the new relationship?

3. The success rate for reversal of laparoscopic sterilization is 25% if performed without the aid of a microscope and as high as 70% with a microscope.

4. The cost of the procedure is £2500 and availability on the NHS is limited. An alternative option would be to consider *in-vitro* fertilization (IVF).

Station 13: Answers

1. The five signs assessed in Apgar scoring are heart rate (beats per minute), respiratory effort, muscle tone, reflex irritability and colour.

2. These parameters are assessed at 1 and 5 minutes.

3. The two actions to resuscitate the baby are to apply oxygen via a bag-valve mask and call the Paediatric Flying Squad.

4. According to the Neonatal Advanced Life Support Protocol, ventilate the baby at 40–60 breaths per minute for 30 seconds with bilateral chest expansion, bilateral breath sounds and adequate colour. Reassess heart rate and the presence of spontaneous respirations. Proceed to endotracheal intubation if this method fails, if there is thick meconium or for prolonged positive-pressure ventilation.

5. For a heart rate < 60 or between 60 and 80 bpm and not climbing, chest compressions are indicated at a 3:1 compression:ventilation ratio or 120 per minute. Depress the sternum by one-third and cease when the heart rate is > 80 bpm.

1. The patient has secondary arrest of cervical dilatation in the first stage of labour.

2. Causes for this arrest include cephalopelvic disproportion, occipotoposterior or occipitotransverse fetal position, or malposition/deflexed fetal head.

3. The next step is to augment her contractions with syntocinon.

4. If labour fails to progress, proceed to a Caesarean section.

5. If the mother was a multigravida, there would be a lower threshold for Caesarean section, and only 4 hours would be given for the mother to show signs of cervical dilatation.

6. Intervention is advised if the cervix continues to efface but not dilate for > 2 hours to the right of the expected line of progression.

7. This condition is called prolonged latent phase of labour. Intervention takes the form of artificial rupture of membranes (ARM) and syntocinon infusion. If the cervix fails to dilate after 4–8 hours, proceed to a Caesarean section.

Station 15: Answers

1. Causes of genuine stress incontinence include pregnancy, vaginal delivery, menopause, previous incontinence surgery or congenital weakness (Ehlers–Danlos syndrome).

2. Treatment for stress incontinence may be divided into medical or surgical. The medical forms of treatment include pelvic floor exercises, oestrogen, vaginal cones and weight loss. Surgical treatment includes TVT or colposuspension, which has an 80–90% success rate at 15 years!

3. Causes of detrusor instability include idiopathic, psychogenic, following incontinence surgery or UMN lesion.

4. Treatment for detrusor instability may also be divided into medical or surgical. Medical treatment includes drug therapy with anticholinergic drugs such as tolteridine (1 mg o bd, increase as required) or oxybutinin XL (od and has fewer side-effects than the former oxybutinin). Other forms of treatment include bladder drill psychotherapy to space apart periods of continence, biofeedback, hypnotherapy, acupuncture, cysto-distension, phenol injections, vaginal denervation procedures and, if the patient is totally desperate, bladder transection, cystoplasty or sacral neurectomy.

This is a favourite DRCOG OSCE topic.

1. The ultrasound indicates a 20-week fetus with symmetric intrauterine growth retardation (IUGR). The HC and AC of the fetus are < 10th percentile and symmetric.

2. Causes of symmetric IUGR include chromosomal abnormalities, congenital infections (cytomegalovirus, parvovirus, rubella, syphilis, toxoplasmosis), race (Asian), sex (female), maternal size, malnutrition and drug abuse (alcohol, tobacco, heroin, methadone).

3. The two investigations you would arrange are chromosomal karyotyping from a fetal blood sample obtained from the umbilical cord at cordocentesis and a maternal screen for the above infections.

4. Fetal well-being may be monitored by the biophysical profile (fetal movements, fetal breathing movements, fetal tone, amniotic fluid volume, fetal cardiotocograph), by the cardiotocograph alone and by Doppler waveform studies of the fetal circulation.

Station 17: Answers

1. Cervical screening is aimed at the 20–65-year-old age group and is offered every 3 years.

2. The smear should ideally be taken mid-cycle. The patient should be advised to avoid a bath on the day, avoid oestrogen creams on the day and abstain from sex for 48 hours before the test.

3. The risk factors for cervical cancer include early coitus, low socio-economic class, multiple sex partners, infection with human papilloma virus (HPV16, 18 and 31), smoking, combined oral contraceptive (coc), childbearing (trauma to the cervix) and chronic cervicitis.

4. According to the cervical screening programme, indications for referral for colposcopy include a borderline cervical smear test on two or three occasions, mild dyskaryosis on two occasions, moderate dyskaryosis on one occasion or severe dyskaryosis on one occasion.

5. Methods of treatment of cervical intraepithelial neoplasia (CIN) include local destructive therapy (CO_2 laser ablation, 'cold' coagulation, cryosurgery, electrocoagulation), local excision (knife cone biopsy, laser cone biopsy, large loop excision of the transformation zone (LLETZ)) and, rarely, hysterectomy.

Station 18: Answers

1. Possible causes for her breakthrough bleeding include the enzyme-inducing effect of carbamazepine on logynon, vomiting or diarrhoea, malabsorption, irregular pill usage, cervical infection or neoplasia.

2. Other enzyme inducers include other anticonvulsants (barbiturates, modafinil, phenytoin, primidone, topiramate), antituberculosis therapy (rifampicin, rifabutin), antifungal (griseofulvin), anti-HIV (ritonavir, nelfinavir, nevirapine), and a proton pump inhibitor (lansoprazole).

3. The patient's options are: carry on with the combined oral contraceptive (coc) pill (use > 50 µg ethinylestradiol-containing coc, a tricyclic preparation or shorten the pill-free interval to 5 days); use Depo-Provera or Noristerat injectables (shorten the period between injections by 2 weeks); use the IUD; consider sterilization or use the barrier method. Options not suitable for her include implanon and the progestogen-only pill.

4. If she should conceive in the future, the patient should be advised to start taking 5 mg folic acid od in early pregnancy as women on carbamazepine or sodium valproate are at increased risk of fetal neural tube defects. Note that if the patient should require emergency contraception in the future, she will need double the dose or two tablets of Levonelle-2 bd as she is on an enzyme-inducer drug.

Station 19: Answers

This is a favourite DRCOG OSCE topic.

1. Yes, she is a candidate. Potential pill failure occurs if two or more pills have been missed from the first seven in a packet or if four or more pills have been missed mid-packet.

2. According to the Faculty of Family Planning (FFP) and the Royal College of Obstetricians and Gynaecologists' guidelines, if two or more combined pills are missed from the last seven pills in a packet, emergency contraception is not required, provided that the pill-free break is omitted. The woman starts her next packet of pills the day after completing the current packet.

3. According to the British Medical Association (BMA)'s Confidentiality and People Under 16 Guidelines, yes, she can legally give consent for medical treatment.

4. The patient should be offered two tablets of Levonelle-2 (one tablet containing 750 mcg levonorgestrel every 12 hours) and domperidone maleate 10 mg to counter nausea and vomiting. The pills are ineffective if vomiting has occurred within 3 hours of ingestion. She should be advised to take the last missed pill in her packet, continue with the packet and use condoms for the next 7 days.

5. As sexual intercourse took place > 72 hours ago, she is not a candidate for the emergency contraceptive pill. Establish that she is not pregnant and discuss fitting the IUD. The IUD is usually inserted within 5 days of unprotected sexual intercourse but may be inserted up to 5 days after the calculated earliest day of ovulation. In this case, unprotected sexual intercourse occurred before ovulation and > 5 days earlier. According to the FFP Guidelines, the IUD may still be inserted.

6. The IUD works by inhibiting implantation and may be inserted at any time in the menstrual cycle.

1. Before prescribing the combined oral contraceptive (coc) pill, you need to know whether the patient is breast-feeding. The coc is contraindicated when breast-feeding. The progestogen-only pill should be offered instead.

2. The coc should be commenced 21 days postpartum.

3. The choices for contraception in breast-feeding mothers are the progestogen-only pill, the lactational amenorrhoea method, Depo-Provera injectable (6 weeks postpartum), the Mirena levonorgestrel intrauterine system (6 weeks postpartum to avoid early expulsion), and barrier methods and spermicides (diaphragms and caps after 6 weeks postpartum). Implanon is contraindicated during breast-feeding.

4. The progestogen-only pill may be started immediately. The patient should be advised to use a condom for the first 7 days. If she has had unprotected sexual intercourse in the past 3 weeks, she should have a urine pregnancy test. However, it takes 2 weeks for the test to turn positive. Consider if she requires emergency contraception.

5. Depo-Provera 150 mg intramuscularly may be administered within the first 5 days of the procedure.